Perfect Medical Presentations

Creating effective PowerPoint presentations for the healthcare professional

Terry Irwin

Director of Gastrointestinal and Endocrine Medicine and Surgery,
Consultant Surgeon, Royal Victoria Hospital, Belfast, UK

Julie Terberg

Owner and principal, Terberg Design, Livonia, Michigan, USA

Foreword by
Geoffrey Glazer

Honorary Consultant Surgeon, St Mary's Hospital, London, UK

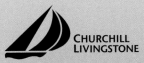

CHURCHILL
LIVINGSTONE

EDINBURGH LONDON NEW YORK OXFORD PHILADELPHIA ST LOUIS SYDNEY TORONTO 2004

CHURCHILL LIVINGSTONE
An imprint of Elsevier Limited

First published 2004

ISBN 0443 074852

British Library Cataloguing in Publication Data
A catalogue record for this book is available from the British Library

Library of Congress Cataloging in Publication Data
A catalog record for this book is available from the Library of Congress

Notice
Medical knowledge is constantly changing. Standard safety precautions must be followed, but as new research and clinical experience broaden our knowledge, changes in treatment and drug therapy may become necessary or appropriate. Readers are advised to check the most current product information provided by the manufacturer of each drug to be administered to verify the recommended dose, the method and duration of administration, and contraindications. It is the responsibility of the practitioner, relying on experience and knowledge of the patient, to determine dosages and the best treatment for each individual patient. Neither the Publisher nor the authors assume any liability for any injury and/or damage to persons or property arising from this publication.

The Publisher

The
Publisher's
policy is to use
**paper manufactured
from sustainable forests**

Printed in China

Contents

About the authors

Terry Irwin
Terry Irwin is a Consultant Colorectal Surgeon at the Royal Victoria Hospital, Belfast, Northern Ireland and an Honorary Lecturer in Surgery to the Queen's University, Belfast, Northern Ireland. He is an experienced postgraduate examiner and previously regional adviser to the Royal College of Surgeons of England. He has extensive experience using and teaching PowerPoint® and digital imaging in medicine. In addition he has authored over 50 publications in major journals.

He set up one of the first websites for surgical trainees in the UK in 1991 and currently designs and manages several professional websites, as well as the one supporting this book.

Julie Terberg
Julie Terberg is the owner and principal of Terberg Design, located in Michigan, which specializes in presentation design and development.

The American Society of Business Publications recently awarded her a gold medal Editor's Choice award in recognition of her Creative Techniques columns, published in Presentations Magazine. She has a BA in Industrial Design from the College for Creative Studies in Detroit, and has been actively involved with computer graphics and presentations since the mid-1980s. She teaches presentation design techniques both in-person and on-line.

Ian Bickle
Ian Bickle is a Senior House Officer in the Royal Victoria Hospital, Belfast, Northern Ireland, with a particular interest in medical writing. He has already co-authored several medical textbooks, including *Clinical Skills for Medical Students* and *Crash Course: Imaging*.

Charles Oppenheim
Charles Oppenheim is Professor of Information Science at Loughborough University, UK. He is the author of *The Legal and Regulatory Environment for Electronic Information*. He is a leading expert on copyright law and data protection.

Joe Niamtu III
Joe Niamtu performed his internship at Carolinas Medical Center in Charlotte, NC and his Oral and Maxillofacial Surgery residency at the Medical College of Virginia.

Dr Niamtu is the chairman of the American Association of Oral and Maxillofacial Surgeons Clinical Interest Group on Cosmetic Surgery. He lectures nationally on various cosmetic facial surgery topics, has edited a textbook on *Cosmetic Facial Surgery*, and contributed chapters in several other international textbooks.

He has written extensively on the use of PowerPoint in medicine and has developed a database for image storage and retrieval.

Jason J Smith

Jason Smith is a Specialist in Colorectal Surgery and is Resident Surgical Officer at St Mark's Hospital, Harrow, UK. He is a tutor in medical informatics for the Royal College of Surgeons of Edinburgh.

He has extensive experience in website design and designs and maintains several websites for surgical societies.

Bob Zeman

Bob Zeman is Chairman of the Department of Radiology and Professor of Radiology at The George Washington University in the USA. He has published on architectural and ergonomic aspects of radiological workstations and on systems for reading DICOM images on Macintosh computers.

R J Winder

John Winder trained as a medical physicist and is currently Lecturer in Medical Imaging at the University of Ulster in Northern Ireland. He lectures on CT, MRI and other aspects of radiological imaging.

John A Carr

Photographer, The Royal College of Surgeons of England, London, UK.

Foreword

Public speaking and presentations – whether for scientific, educational, commercial or other purposes – has entered a new dimension. The old techniques of the blackboard and chalk, the flip chart, or the overhead projector and a set of coloured pencils are almost, but not quite, dead. For those more attuned to glass slides (which will include most readers) and Letraset (that time-consuming method of stencilling and hand drawing slides) the electronic era has brought a degree of trepidation.

It's not that these steam-age techniques were fault free, far from it. Most amateurs, like myself, will recall the terrors of the slide projectors. Slides mysteriously appeared upside down or on their side and then came the dreaded jamming of the carousel, after which a helpful member of the audience would leap to the rescue and, turning everything upside down, would tip all the slides into an uncoordinated heap. Sometimes the slides seemed to melt and warp before a mesmerized audience, and now and then an ominous crack spread across the glass like a bolt of lightning, scarring the landscape of the most prized and important slide. On one occasion, at an international meeting attended by one of the authors of this book, I was the victim of a manic projector, which suddenly erupted and belched my slides into the air one after another. This particular presentation ended abruptly at this point, with the audience convulsed in hysterics and all going out for an early coffee break.

I doubt that this farcical event was the major stimulus to this book but rather the fact that the authors were aware of the new difficulties and dangers of PowerPoint® presentations. Now, as we arrive at a conference we see speakers struggling with an unresponsive computer and watch with morbid fascination as they furiously and impotently click on their 'A' disc or CD-ROM. Sometimes we see the overconfident expert walk to the podium with his personal laptop that cannot be connected with the projector. Too often the speaker presses the wrong key and we are plunged into an electronic void or, worst still, back to the beginning of an already tedious talk. Even if there is mastery of the technology, the presentation might be too wordy; or set-up in bland, unreadable colours; or the special effects of funny photos, moving bullet points, videos and sound effects distract from the main thrust of the presentation. 'The PowerPoint is the Message' to paraphrase Marshall McLuhan.

Terry Irwin and Julie Terberg have written a remarkably readable and practical book to help beginners and aficionados to understand and improve their computer presentations. I will not reiterate here all the topics covered but they include some of the important legal aspects of public presentations, as well as the general and fine detail of PowerPoint. I congratulate them on this thoughtful and knowledgeable book, and I am sure readers will find plenty here to educate and amuse them.

One final word to all electronic enthusiasts, in which category I place myself. Let us not forget the beauty and power of the English language, which can be so brutalized by computer presentations. This has been illustrated by the recent publication of the Gettysburg address alongside a PowerPoint template presentation of the same, which shows that even this eloquent and moving speech can be reduced to nonsensical jargon. PowerPoint enthusiasts – take note!

Geoffrey Glazer MS FRCS FACS
Honorary Consultant Surgeon,
St Mary's Hospital,
Praed Street,
London W2
2004

Preface

If you are a healthcare professional, whether a doctor, dentist, nurse or scientist *and* you give lectures or tutorials this book is for you. Even if you are an experienced presenter, we expect that you will find lots of useful tips that will improve your presentations. We take you from important basic knowledge about digital images in medical presentations, right through to instructions for putting a presentation together. Indeed we also deal with how to give the presentation itself, because content is only part of getting your message across.

We have found that most healthcare professionals are familiar with a presentation package such as Microsoft PowerPoint®, but use only a fraction of the potential of the program. There are many additional features of PowerPoint that can enhance a presentation and that are easy to learn.

If you are a beginner, perhaps intimidated by PowerPoint, we will walk you step by step from opening the program to presenting superb looking talks in a matter of an hour or two. You will even learn how to make your own PowerPoint templates.

You will want to add images to your presentation, but many people find this confusing. It should be possible to produce a PowerPoint presentation containing half a dozen high quality images and still keep the total file size less than one megabyte. If you do not know how to do this, this book is definitely for you. We will explain what image file types mean, how you choose the correct one for each situation and why this is important.

The most recent innovation for medical teachers has been the advent of digital imaging. We use the term imaging rather than photography, because a scan of an X-ray is an image, not a photograph, but you can consider the terms synonymous if you like. Lack of understanding of image formats causes endless problems, usually because huge files are generated by the unsuspecting.

Modern radiology departments are digital, of course, lending them to the capture of radiology images directly from the system without the need to scan hard copies. The chapter on digital radiological images will explain how such systems work and how to extract images directly from them.

One of the most important issues that this book addresses is consent. Recent guidelines have clarified the rules in many countries and we will give guidance on what consent means and how to protect your images and yourself.

It is always easier to learn by doing rather than reading. All the files that you need to complete the exercises in this book are included on the CD in the back cover, along with a trial copy of Adobe's award winning program Photoshop Elements®.

OK. I've got ten minutes.
How do I use PowerPoint?

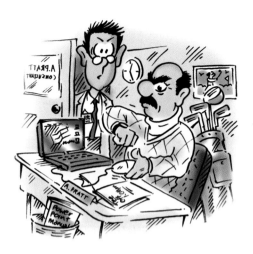

Each chapter in the book should take about one hour to read. They can be read in any order, but we strongly recommend that you start with the first few chapters so that you understand the basics. By the time you have read the whole book, you will be able to produce stunning PowerPoint presentations that don't cause your laptop to fall over with exhaustion. Along the way we hope that you find the exercises fun.

We have used some conventions throughout the book, which we hope will make it easier to follow the instructions. Basic text is formatted as in this preface. Commands – that is, a series of selections from the menu of either PowerPoint or Photoshop Elements – are formatted like this:

Insert>Picture>From File where each word or phrase separated by a ">" represents a choice on a menu. Hints and reminders are indicated with '!!!!!! Note!' in the margin.

We have used US English throughout the book. We hope that UK readers in particular will forgive this, especially since one of us is a surgeon practicing in the UK, but we had to make a decision to use a consistent style throughout.

The book is supported by a website, which you can find at www.perfectmedicalpresentations.com. We cannot provide formal support to every reader, but the website includes further information, links and downloads. Most importantly, there is a bulletin board where you can post questions or let us know about errors or omissions. If we ever manage to produce a second edition, the comments on the website will be very important to us. We may just reward the most helpful bulletin board members with a copy of the second edition!

Terry Irwin and
Julie Terberg, 2004

Acknowledgements

This book was inspired by the difficulties that many colleagues have faced with presentations. We hope that it will be of some help to them in the future.

In 1832 Morse wrote that he saw 'no reason why intelligence may not be transmitted instantaneously by electricity to any distance'.

The two authors have never met, nor spoken to each other on the telephone! The fact that we were able to find each other, agree to produce this book and collaborate fully in its production is a testament to the power of electronic communication and proof that Morse was right.

We are grateful to the many people who have offered much needed help. In particular, most of the beautiful images were supplied by John Carr, photographer to the Royal College of Surgeons of England to whom we owe a debt of gratitude.

Comments on individual chapters were received from Dr Ross Boardman, Dr Derek Kelly and Dr Kathleen Singlott (fellow students on the Diploma in Medical Informatics course at the Royal College of Surgeons of Edinburgh), Irene Dworakowski (American College of Surgeons), Dr Bill Smyth (Medical Protection Society, UK), Graham Partin (Australian Medical Council), Pamela Burton (Australian Medical Association). While these individuals gave much valued advice, they are not in any way responsible for any errors or omissions on our part.

Drawings were produced by the talented Andras Barabas, (author of an excellent book on medical presentations, now sadly out of print) and Johnny Simms.

This has been a labor of love for both of us. We are indebted to our better halves, Jenny Irwin and Bob Terberg who put up with our obsession.

The book is dedicated to our children, Sarah, Sam and Charlotte Irwin and Jacob and Megan Terberg. They will all be much better than us at this before we know or acknowledge it.

Terry Irwin and
Julie Terberg, 2004

Chapter 1

The history of digital imaging in medicine

Ian Bickle and Terry Irwin

Digital images are an integral part of medical science. Whether you are talking about a magnetic resonance (MR) scan, an image in a PowerPoint® presentation or a video clip of a patient, we have come to accept that they are part of what we do. It is hard to remember a time when we did not use digital images but in fact it is much less than a decade since they became commonplace.

On 25 May 1961, the President of the United States, John F. Kennedy, told the world 'I believe that this nation should commit itself to achieving the goal, before this decade is out, of landing a man on the moon and returning him safely to the earth'. Little did anyone appreciate that as a result not only would we be able fry an egg without it sticking to the pan but that we would reap the benefits of digital imaging in medicine.

Long before Neill Armstrong and Buzz Aldrin set foot on the moon in 1969, the National Aeronautical and Space Association (NASA) was exploring the moon's surface as part of its preparation for the manned Apollo missions that would follow. Indeed, as early as 1959 the first unmanned Ranger mission took close up images of the moon's surface. A substantive element of these NASA missions of the early 1960s was the Lunar Orbiter Program. The prime purpose of this program was to acquire high-resolution images of the surface of the moon so that suitable landing sites for the Apollo and Surveyor spacecraft could be identified. Acquiring images vast distances from earth without direct human input proved an immense challenge.

The initial Ranger missions had attempted to broadcast analog signals from transmitters outfitted to video cameras but conventional receivers were unable to transform them into clear images because of interference from natural radio sources. NASA's Jet Propulsion Laboratory set about solving this problem. This involved the use of computer technology, then in its infancy, to improve the analog signals by processing them into numerical (or digital) information. This rather crude process of digitization allowed interference to be removed.

By the Block III Ranger missions in 1964/5, clear images were being acquired, allowing careful planning of potential landing sites and ultimately for Apollo 11 to land on the Moon on 20 July 1969.

Two of the pioneers involved in the development of digital imaging were George Smith and William Boyle at Bell Laboratories. Together they developed the charge-coupled device (CCD) in 1969. This light-sensitive circuit can hold data as a charge. This is then passed through an amplifier and analog-to-digital converter to produce digital signals. The CCD is now the basis of all digital cameras and a host of electronic devices ranging from camcorders to medical imaging equipment.

In 1972 the British engineer (later Sir) Godfrey Hounsfield of EMI Laboratories developed computerized axial tomography CAT (later shortened to CT) based on this new digital computer technology. The Nobel Peace Prize winner's work first came into the clinical arena in 1974. Widespread full-body CT was available by the 1980s, offering a new tool in the diagnosis of medical illness. The slices (axial images) were stored digitally on computer and could then be reconstructed, offering previously unheard of 'pictures' of transverse sectional anatomy.

In the early 1980s digital subtraction angiography, which utilized analog-to-digital converters and computers to allow accurate visualization of arteries while subtracting background data, replaced the older and much clumsier technique of taking a positive and a negative image (only one of which contained contrast) and subtracting one from the other by exposing a third plate under both of these.

Spiral CT was developed in 1989 – now offering continuous data acquisition, rather than the 'stop–start' process of the original scanners. Today, CT has developed further offering 16 multi-slice scanners capable of producing forty slices in as many seconds. New applications such as CT angiography are made possible by reconstructing these image slices in a variety of planes.

Paul Lauterbus at Thorn-EMI led the development of magnetic resonance imaging (MRI) and took this new imaging from research in the 1970s to commercial use in medicine by 1984 – only expense preventing it becoming mainstream until the 1990s.

In addition to these new technologies, conventional radiological imaging techniques were upgraded to digital from analogue. This in itself has many advantages to the user. Perhaps most importantly it allows images to be accessed via computers networked throughout a hospital or further afield. Multiple users can access, interpret, and manipulate images at any one time using systems such as the picture archiving and communication system (PACS).

In parallel with the advances in radiological imaging came advances in camera technology. The digital camera has captivated a whole generation and it seems few families are now without one; they are now commonplace in hospitals and general practice surgeries.

Telemedicine was a further development of the 'space age'. During manned missions, NASA recorded physiological measurements from its astronauts. This data was analyzed on earth while the mission continued. NASA was integral in funding some of the original telemedicine projects. STARPAHC (Space Technology Applied to Rural Papago Advanced Health Care) looked at ways of delivering healthcare to the Papago Indian Reservation in Arizona. Remote settlements could now have immediate access to expertise to assist with life-and-death decisions in medical emergencies.

Digital images are now routinely used to send information about patients from one location to another. This might take the form of still images, as in teledermatology projects, or moving images in remote fetal ultrasound reporting. Some of this is synchronous, where the sender and viewer see the images together, in real time. Some is asynchronous, where an opinion is generated and returned at a later time. All of it offers potential benefits if used appropriately.

The problem has been that while many of us have grasped this new technology, few of us really understand how to use it! All too often we see presentations fail because the author has tried to incorporate digital information such as images or video without understanding how to compress them to manageable size.

Imagine what doctors and nurses in 1961 would have thought of all of this? You may never look at the moon in the same light again!

Chapter 2

What is a digital image?

Terry Irwin and Julie Terberg

Although this is not a technical manual, it is important to understand a little bit about how a computer codes for color. Ironically, if you are unfamiliar with this you might feel that it is not important to you. However, as you begin to understand how color works in a computer, you will see why it helps to have a basic knowledge. Don't worry though; we won't get bogged down in detail.

An image on a computer is composed of a series of dots, called pixels (short for 'picture elements'). Just think of how a tapestry is created using individual stitches of different colored thread (Fig. 2.1). On a computer, each dot of color has a unique reference number that tells the computer what color it is. It also carries information about where it is (its *x* and *y* coordinates, but we can safely ignore this).

A bit is a single item of information in a computer. Computers use binary code – on or off, one or zero. If you use 8 bits (one byte) to describe a color, the largest resulting binary number will be eight digits long, each of which will be a 1 or a 0, such as: 11010111. The largest number you can describe with this method is 11111111. This is the number 255 in our decimal notation.

Figure 2.1
A tapestry looks like a picture from a distance, but up close the individual stitches are visible.

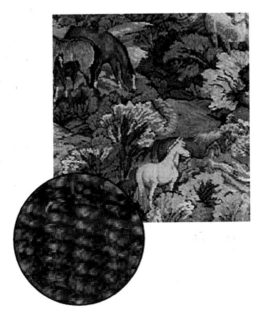

If you don't believe this, open the calculator on your computer, switch to scientific mode (View > Scientific) and type in '255'. Now switch to binary mode by tapping the radio button 'Bin' (Fig. 2.2).

You can also have a color defined as 00000000, zero in the more familiar decimal notation, which is black. So the choice of colors is from 00000000 (black) to 11111111 (white) and a total of 256 individual colors can be coded for using this system.

Figure 2.2
11111111 really is 255!

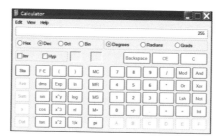

Some image files will be coded using 256 colors, typically graphics interchange format (GIF). We will explain later why you need to understand that a GIF has only 256 possible colors, but for now just think how many colors there are in a high-quality photographic image and what it might look like if you had only 256 to choose from. For some images, 256 colors just will not do (Fig. 2.3)!

Figure 2.3
Sometimes 256 colors just isn't enough!

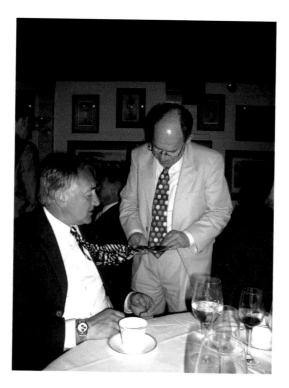

Contemporary computer monitors can display millions of colors. Nearly every monitor sold today supports superVGA (SVGA) mode, which is defined as a 24-bit display. With a 24-bit display, 8 bits of memory are dedicated to each of the three additive primary colors: red, green, and blue (8 + 8 + 8 = 24). This is also called 'true color' because it can produce more than the 10 million colors discernable to the human eye. Think of each pixel as being made up of three monochromatic layers, the red layer will consist of any one of 256 values of red, the green layer any one of 256 values of green, and the blue layer any one of 256 values of blue. The final composite color will be any one of 256 times 256 times 256, or about 16.8 million different color combinations.

Display mode

Your monitor may be capable of displaying 32-bit (true color). This is a special graphics mode used by digital video, animation, and video games to achieve certain effects. Essentially, 24 bits are used for color and the other 8 bits are used as a separate layer for representing levels of translucency in an object or image.

Additive colors

A monitor uses red, green, and blue (RGB) light to create colors. Combining or 'adding' full intensities of all three colors makes white. Your computer monitor, for example, creates color by emitting light through red, green, and blue phosphors (Fig. 2.4).

When you take a digital photograph, or scan an X-ray, you are creating a file composed of pixels, where each pixel's position on the screen (its x and y position) and its color are coded using this system. You will need to decide whether the information contained in the image can be described in 256 colors without loss of clarity (possibly a black and white line diagram) or whether 16 million colors are needed. We will explain how to make this decision later.

Do you really need to know this? Well, take an X-ray as an example. This is composed of a tonal range of grays, from white to black. It contains no colors. If you scan it as a color image rather than as a grayscale image, you will end up with a file three times larger than you need. On the other hand, a line drawing contains only black or white. If you scan it incorrectly, you will end up with a file many hundreds of times bigger than you need.

Figure 2.4
Think of an image as a combination of the three primary colors.

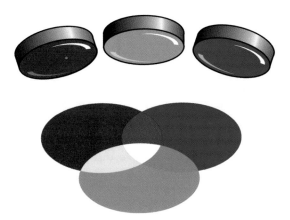

Your digital camera takes images using a charge coupled device (CCD; see Chapter 1). This is a series of photosensitive elements, each of which records one pixel of information. A three-megapixel (mega = million) camera will record three million dots, each represented by 3 bytes (remember, each pixel is coded using 3 bytes: one for each of red, green, and blue). Thus the image will be at least 9 megabytes in size if it is not compressed.

Thankfully, digital cameras use compression; usually saving the image as a jpeg file (we will describe file formats in the next chapter). None the less, on a standard 3-megapixel camera, each image captured at high resolution will be at least 1 megabyte in size. This is a huge file to insert into a PowerPoint® presentation and it will need to be 'optimized' to ensure that your computer loads the images quickly (we will cover this later, too).

Your monitor can be set to display the screen area at different pixel ratios. The most common display settings are 800 × 600 and 1024 × 768. The digital image from your 3-megapixel camera, when viewed on your computer screen, will have about 2500 pixels along its horizontal axis (and 1200 vertically). If you do not make the image smaller, it will be bigger than the screen!

Many of you who have tried to put a digital image directly from your camera into PowerPoint will at this point be saying 'Ah, that explains why it does that'. Furthermore, all those extra pixels are using up memory. You need to reduce the size of the image so that it fits on the screen and does not contain more pixels than the screen can display. This will substantially reduce the file size, but only if you do it correctly. If you just grab the corner of the image and drag it smaller the file size remains the same, it is only the visible area of image that is smaller. Yes, we will teach you how to do this in a later chapter as well!

Let's go back to our tapestry model for understanding pixels. If you look at a tapestry from the far side of a room it looks like an image. If you walk right up to it and look very closely, you can see the individual stitches. Similarly, if you continue to magnify a digital image, after a while you can begin to make out the individual pixels. The image starts to 'pixilate' (Fig. 2.5).

This is an important concept to understand for digital image storage. You can make digital images bigger, but if you increase the size by more than 150% the pixilation will begin to show. You can use image manipulation software to enlarge the image and the program will add in extra pixels to fill in those that are missing, sampling nearby pixels to select color. However, this method eventually produces a blurred image (Fig. 2.6).

The practical importance of this is that you should always store the original image in its unaltered form before you make any changes to it. It is best to save it as an uncompressed file such as a .tiff, .psd, or .bmp file. Saving it as a jpeg might be OK but jpeg files are compressed using a system called lossy compression and the more you compress, the more quality is lost. You will learn later that you should store the original image and make any size, shape, or color changes to a duplicate image. Never change your master image; you might eventually need to use the original for another purpose.

Let's say, for example, that you take a picture of a patient and reduce it in size and compress it (as a .jpeg) for use on the web. The picture might now be 150 × 100 pixels and a nice small file that will download easily. You subsequently decide to produce a poster for a meeting and you want to use

Figure 2.5
Any image will pixilate if enlarged too much.

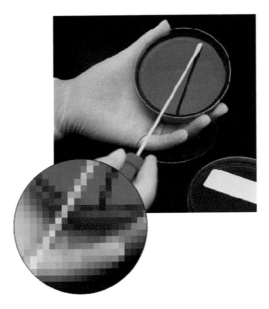

Figure 2.6
Image manipulation software fills in extra pixels when a small image is enlarged, producing blurred results.

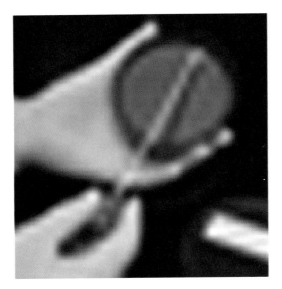

the same image at a size of 6 inches by 4 inches. The image can be enlarged again but it now has only 25 pixels per inch and will look terrible. Had you stored the original image (remember the digital camera image was 2500 pixels across) it would print at over 400 pixels per inch (2500 pixels in 6 inches is equivalent to 416 pixels per inch), which is as good as a photograph in a book. The images in this book are printed at 300 pixels per inch.

If this is all beginning to worry you – relax. All of these issues will be covered step by step in this book. If you are beginning to recognize that you have experienced these sorts of problems, read on!

Chapter 3

Choosing the correct file format

Terry Irwin and Julie Terberg

The quality of the images that you produce depends almost as much on how you save them as it does on the actual image. Most people are familiar with the .jpeg format and presume that it is the correct format to save images for all purposes. Nothing could be further from the truth. The problem is that once you have saved an image in an incorrect format, it may be lost forever.

A number of images are included on the companion CD. Start Photoshop Elements®, and open the file 'sample.tif' located in the Chapter 3 folder.

! ! ! ! ! ! ! ! ! ! ! ! ! ! ! ! ! *Note !*

A trial (tryout) version of Photoshop Elements is provided on the companion CD. You can use this version to follow along with the examples. Alternatively, you might prefer to use another image manipulation program such as the full version of Adobe Photoshop®, Paintshop Pro®, Corel PhotoPaint® or another you are familiar with.

'Sample.tif' looks like a reasonable image of a patient but there is quite a lot of unnecessary space around the edges and the image is not square (Fig. 3.1). In this instance, you can always refer to the original file on the CD, therefore you do not need to save a copy before making any revisions.

Figure 3.1
Patient.tif

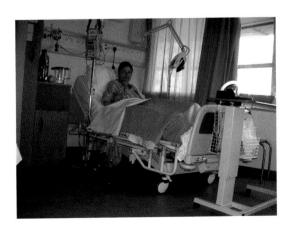

Figure 3.2
The crop tool.

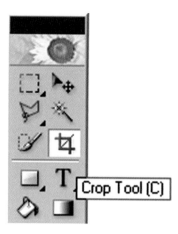

Select View > Fit on screen (Ctrl 0) to see the whole image. We want to get rid of the excess image around the outside.

Select the crop tool (Fig. 3.2) and draw a rectangle on the image approximately where you wish to crop. Notice the 'shield' on the toolbar at the top of your screen. If you check the 'shield' tick-box the rest of the image will darken, making it easier to see what you are doing. You can move the crop box about by clicking inside the dashed rectangle and holding down the mouse button while moving it around (drag). Select any one of the 'handles' on the rectangle to resize your crop selection. If you move the cursor a slight distance away from the handles, you will see a rotation handle: an arc with two arrows. Click and drag on this rotation handle to freely rotate the selection (Fig. 3.3).

Figure 3.3
Preparing to crop the image.

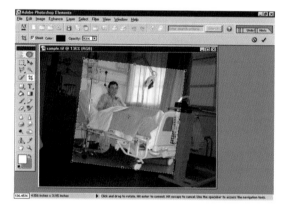

As a guide, the drip stand and the edge of the locker ought to be vertical, so make sure the edge of your crop box is parallel with these.

When you are satisfied with the image, hit 'Enter'.

You should now have a straight image that does not contain any clutter. Note that the drip stand is vertical (Fig. 3.4).

Save the file immediately. Select File > Save As and select a safe folder for storage. Rename the file 'patient' and use the drop-down arrow to select 'TIFF' under the 'Format' option. This is your master file and you should never

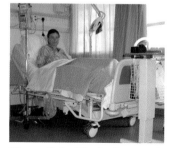

Figure 3.4   The final cropped image.

replace or change it. Any further changes to the image must be saved under a different file name.

Before we explore file types you need to be aware of two terms that will recur throughout this book: 'layers' and 'transparency'.

Layers

Imagine a drawing on a sheet of acetate, say, an anatomical image. You want to add labels to the image that you can overlay and remove. You might do this by drawing the labels on a second acetate sheet. When you want to show the image with the labels you can put one sheet on top of the other and project both. Similarly, in Photoshop Elements you can construct layers, which you can choose to be visible or hidden. If you are happy that your image is complete and you will never need to separate the layers again you can merge the layers (Fig. 3.5).

We will explore layers in greater detail in a later chapter, but for now you just need to be aware of the concept.

Figure 3.5
Layers and transparency can be thought of as using acetate sheets, laid one on top of another.

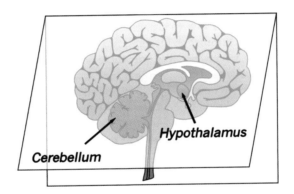

Transparency

Again we will use our acetate model to explain this. In the majority of image types, the whole canvas is composed of color. Quite often, the background is white. When you want to show an image on an overhead projector, you print on acetate, making the 'paper' color transparent. It appears white when projected because the screen color shows through.

Similarly, you might have an image, such as a logo – possibly an irregular shape – that you want to layer on top of a different color or pattern in PowerPoint®. If the background canvas for the logo consists of a solid color, you can attempt to erase the background in PowerPoint.

To follow along with this example, open a new file in PowerPoint. Select Format > Background, click on the drop-down arrow and choose 'More Colors'. Choose a dark blue color swatch; click 'OK' and then 'Apply to all'. If you are a complete novice and have never used PowerPoint, just open the file 'HCS.ppt' from the Chapter 3 folder on the CD.

Select Insert > Picture > From File, choose the file 'HCSlogo.jpg' (from the Chapter 3 folder). If the Picture toolbar does not appear automatically, right-click on the logo and select 'Show Picture Toolbar'. On this toolbar, select the 'Set Transparent Color' icon and click anywhere on the white area surrounding the logo. The resulting logo appears to have a speckled (aliased) edge, especially on the dark blue background (Fig. 3.6).

Figure 3.6
The aliased edge of the logo is distracting in PowerPoint.

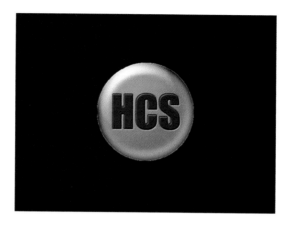

It is easy to change the background so that it is truly transparent. Go back to Photoshop Elements and open the file 'HCSlogo.jpg' (from the CD). If the Layers window is not visible, select Window > Layers. You will need to change the background layer to an editable layer to achieve transparency. Hold down the 'Alt' key and then in the layers window, double-click on the background layer. The layer name will change to 'Layer 0'.

Now we will use the Magic Wand tool. Type 'W' or select the Magic Wand tool from the toolbar (Fig. 3.7). Change the tolerance level on the options toolbar to '25' and then click anywhere in the white background. Marching ants (an animated, dashed line) will appear around the logo. This indicates the white area has been selected. To delete this area, hit the 'Delete' key, type 'Ctrl X', or select Edit > Cut.

Figure 3.7
The Magic Wand tool in Photoshop Elements.

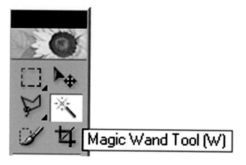

You now have a transparent background – you can tell because of the gray and white checkerboard pattern (Fig. 3.8). This is Photoshop's method of indicating transparency. Select File > Save As, choose .PNG as the format type and name the file 'HCSlogo'. It is important to select the .PNG format because it supports transparency; if you use .JPG you will lose the transparent background.

Now switch to your PowerPoint file, and move the HCS logo to the left. Select Insert > Picture > From File, and navigate to the new file: 'HCSlogo.png'.

Figure 3.8
The logo prepared with a transparent background.

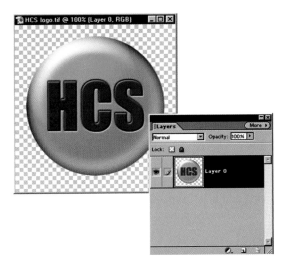

Figure 3.9
Compare the original aliased logo (left) with the anti-aliased logo (right) correctly prepared in Photoshop Elements.

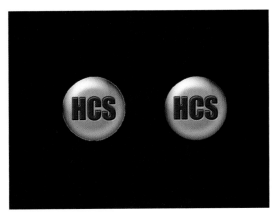

This will insert the logo in the center of the screen; simply drag it to the right for a comparison (Fig. 3.9).

Notice how much cleaner the edge is around the logo. You can achieve the same effect with the logo for your hospital, specialty association or unit, to give a more professional look to your presentation. Later in the book we will teach you how to improve the image further by using some of the simple tricks in Photoshop Elements.

File types

BMP (Windows® Bitmap)

This is a basic file type for many images. This large file type is generally unsuited to manipulation and should not be used in PowerPoint.

GIF (graphics interchange format)

The GIF file format uses only 256 colors and is suitable for simple images only. It is particularly suited to line drawings but is not detailed enough for photographs or other continuous tone images. There are two types of GIF file: The 89a format allows pixels to be transparent, which is why it is often used for logos on the web. GIF files can be animated (made to appear to move). Incidentally, it is pronounced 'JIFF', rather than with a hard G.

For an example of an animated GIF made from a photographic original, using PowerPoint, open 'Sam.ppt' from the Chapter 3 folder on the CD. Hit the 'F5' key to view the slide show (hit the 'Esc' key to exit). This was created with a series of similar photographs, using a free GIF construction program downloaded from the net.

GIF files are usually very small. This is achieved by the method of compression. As there are relatively few colors in the image, there will be large areas of the same color and this area is coded as a unit, rather than as individual pixels. Thus the amount of data needed to describe the image is greatly reduced.

JPEG (joint photographics expert group)

This is a lossy compression file format that can compress images up to 20-fold. This means that a 1-megabyte image can be reduced to 50 000 bytes. You can choose how much compression you want to apply, depending on the final purpose of the image. Each time an image is resaved as a JPEG image it is compressed, and thus image quality gradually degrades. Therefore, the image should be saved as a JPEG file only when it has been cropped, rotated, resized, and so on. This format does not support layers or transparency.

JPEG files are generally very small, so they are ideal for use on the web. They *can* be used for images in PowerPoint but make sure that the image is exactly as you want it to be in terms of size, shape, content, and resolution (we will come to that later) before you save it as a .jpeg for the first and last time.

PNG (portable network graphics)

This file format was developed to replace GIF but in fact it offers many features in common with TIFF and JPEG formats. It allows areas of the image to be transparent and is very useful for saving logos and other complex images using full color. This format works well in PowerPoint.

PSD (native Photoshop file format)

This format can retain information about layers and transparency. Compression is lossless; there is no image degradation. Use this file format to save all of your layers for further editing in Photoshop Elements. PowerPoint does not support this format.

TIFF (tag image file format)

The TIFF format was designed over 25 years ago in an attempt to standardize image formats. TIFF files can be saved in uncompressed form, or using LZW compression (see Chapter 8 for an explanation), which does not cause any loss of quality of the image and reduces the file size by about 50%. TIFF files can also be saved using ZIP or JPEG compression to reduce file size, yet these options may reduce image quality. When saving a TIFF file, you may choose to save layers and transparency. A transparent TIFF file will work in PowerPoint. However, your image size will be substantially larger than that of a PNG file.

Saving your file

When you save a file in Photoshop Elements you will be given a choice of file formats. If this is your final image and it is for use in PowerPoint or on the web, JPEG is usually the correct choice. You will be given a choice of degree of compression as well. The more you compress the image, the smaller the file but the greater the loss of quality. If the file is a complex Photoshop image with layers, PSD is the best choice. If it is a simple line drawing choose GIF. If it is the original image and you need to preserve quality, choose TIFF.

Image degradation

In Photoshop Elements, re-open the file 'patient.tif' that you saved at the start of this chapter. Remember to save it as a different file in each of these exercises!

Select File > Save As, and select the JPEG format. When prompted to select the image quality, choose 'Low quality (maximum compression)' by moving the sliding handle to the left. Notice how much smaller the file size is. You should be able to reduce it from the original 12 megabytes down to just over 122 kilobytes at a quality level of '1'. This is a very large initial image, taken with a 6-megapixel camera, so the loss of quality is not very obvious. Plus, you have saved it only once.

These examples are of a close-up of the face from the original TIFF file and then in a JPEG that has been saved five times. There has been a significant loss of quality (Fig. 3.10).

Figure 3.10
When this image is saved five times as a JPEG there is significant loss of quality.

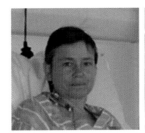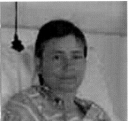

By now you should have an understanding of the different file types commonly used in Photoshop Elements and which file format you would choose for a particular task.

Chapter 4

Resolution explained

Terry Irwin and Julie Terberg

An understanding of resolution is important if you are to get the best out of your camera, scanner or computer. Resolution affects image quality. On the one hand, if you try to reproduce an image beyond the tolerance of its resolution it will look poor – in digital imaging terms it will 'pixilate'. You have probably downloaded an image from the internet and tried to use it in a Word™ document only to find that it looks very poor, especially when printed. On the other hand, if you have a high-resolution image and show it using equipment that cannot match this resolution, you are wasting disk space and slowing the whole process. You will no doubt have seen someone at a meeting (not you, of course!) running a PowerPoint® presentation that includes at least one image that makes the laptop stall and perhaps quit altogether. Equally, you might have waited an age for an image to download from a web page (a phenomenon known as the 'world wide wait').

Digital cameras cannot yet achieve the resolution of emulsion film. Indeed, the very highest-quality professional digital systems, with over 45 megapixels, still fall short of the quality of emulsion film. Thankfully, for our purposes, this does not matter because we will most often be showing images on a computer screen or data projector, where all this extra resolution is wasted anyway.

Resolution also depends on the viewing distance. Take a look at a photograph in a newspaper. Hold it very close and you can see every dot. Hold it at arms length and you perceive it as a continuous-tone picture. Similarly, a poster on a billboard seen at a distance looks very different from the same image at close range. Resolution depends on the:

- input device (digital camera or scanner)
- output device (computer monitor, data projector or printer)
- viewing distance.

For most purposes you should aim to achieve an image resolution that is sufficient for the weakest link in the chain of input and output devices. Scanning an image at 1200 dots per inch (dpi), from a book that is printed at

300 dpi is just a waste of time and disk space. If you are going to display the image in a presentation or on a website then you should scan it to fit within common screen display sizes. It is really that simple!

!!!!!!!!!!!!!!!!!! Note !

The term dpi – dots per inch – is relevant only when printing. In printing, dpi is the measure of printed image quality on the paper. Pixel dimensions are relevant to all images displayed on a computer. This is sometimes called ppi, or pixels per inch. A high-resolution monitor setting will display more pixels per inch.

Scanning at too high a resolution is called oversampling and is the most common error made in medical imaging. It results in unnecessarily large files (see Chapter 11 for more information about scanning).

Brightness resolution

We explained color depth in Chapter 2 – it refers to the number of colors in the image. Most images have a bit depth of 8, that is, each color channel (red, green, and blue) is coded using 8 bits and the range of colors available is 2^8 or 256 colors per channel, which equates to over 16 million colors. Some authors refer to this as 'brightness resolution'.

We have already explained that images with simple graphics or limited color work well as GIFs rather than JPEGs. Thankfully, Photoshop Elements® allows you to preview your images and their file size before you make any changes.

Remember that grayscale images such as X-rays do not need three channels to convey color information, so you can code them in 256 'colors', which really means 256 variations of black and white. You might find that a color image in your presentation also works well in grayscale, so let's see how easy it is to convert a three-channel, 16 million color image to a single-channel, 256 color image using Photoshop Elements.

Start Photoshop Elements, and open 'lily.tif' from the Chapter 4 folder on the CD. Note that it is about 5 megabytes in size. Now change it to a grayscale image by selecting Image > Mode > Grayscale. You will be asked whether you want to discard the color information – click 'OK'. Select File > Save As, select TIFF format and rename the file 'graylily.tif'. The image is now about 1.63 megabytes (Fig. 4.1), about one-third of the size – no surprise!

When you have read Chapter 11 on scanning images, you will know why and how to scan X-rays in grayscale mode. If you already have files that have been scanned incorrectly in color mode, you can change them using this technique.

Figure 4.1
The original color image is 4.9 megabytes. After removal of color information, the file is one third the size of the full color version.

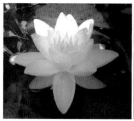 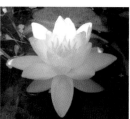

Image resolution

Image resolution is sometimes called spatial resolution and refers to the number of pixels in the image, measured in pixels per inch. A 6-megapixel digital camera will produce images that are roughly 3000 by 2000 pixels.

! ! ! ! ! ! ! ! ! ! ! ! ! ! ! ! Note !

If you have a computer that is getting a bit old or slow, do not try this next exercise. You might regret it!

Open the image 'highresolution.tif' using Photoshop Elements. This is a high-resolution image captured with a 6-megapixel camera. Open the image size dialogue box: select Image > Resize > Image size. Note that the image size is over 14 megabytes. The image measures 2560 pixels by 1920 pixels. This image would be over 35 inches wide if shown on a monitor at 72 dpi. Do you have a 36-inch monitor?

Leave Photoshop Elements open for now and start PowerPoint. On a blank slide select Insert > Picture > From File, navigate to the chapter folder and double-click the file 'flower.jpg'. Note that it is far too big for the slide (Fig. 4.2: we thought we would spare you the operative image and let you play with some images from my garden instead!). Most people would simply drag the corner of the image to make it fit but this leaves the image at the same file size (hope you have a really fast laptop!).

Go back to Photoshop Elements and open the image 'flower.jpg'. We want the image to fit on the PowerPoint screen. Select Image > Resize > Image Size, make sure that 'constrain proportions' is ticked before you change the image size. In the 'Image Size' window, under 'Pixel Dimensions', you will see width and height dimensions. If the dimensions are specified as a percentage, click the drop-down arrows to change these to pixels. Change the number of pixels in width to 400.

! ! ! ! ! ! ! ! ! ! ! ! ! ! ! ! Note !

By default the image dimensions are 'constrained', this means that when the width is increased or decreased the height scales by the same amount.

You'll notice that next to 'Pixel Dimensions' the image size has been reduced to 352 kilobytes. Save the new image as a .jpeg file ('myflower' will do) and see how much smaller it is now. Using minimal compression to retain quality, it reduces to about 211 kilobytes. Yes, you really have reduced a 14-megabyte image to 211 kilobytes without any loss of quality.

Figure 4.2
If not correctly resized, digital images will be significantly larger than the size of your PowerPoint slide.

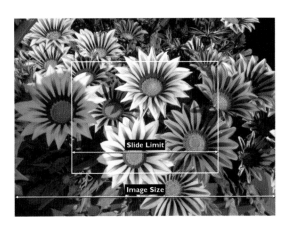

Switch to PowerPoint, choose Insert > Duplicate slide, select the picture and hit 'Delete'. Select Insert > Picture > From File, and then 'myflower.jpg' from your work folder. This new image fits well on the slide. This image should occupy a little over a quarter of the slide area. If you want the image larger, select a higher image width in the image dimensions above when you are resizing the image in Photoshop Elements.

Screen resolution

The other common form of output resolution is screen resolution. The number of pixels displayed across the width of your computer monitor or data projector image is also called the display setting. The most common settings are 800 × 600 and 1024 × 768 (Fig. 4.3).

Figure 4.3
Setting up your display
properties.

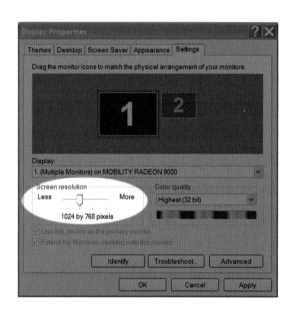

!!!!!!!!!!!!!!!!!!!! Tip !

Check your current display setting in Windows by right-clicking anywhere on your desktop, select Properties > Settings, and note the pixel dimensions indicated for Screen Area. On a Mac: 'Apple Monitor Control Panel'.

Before changing this to a higher setting, make sure your data projector is capable of displaying the higher resolution.

If your display is set for 1024 × 768, images saved at a higher resolution will not project any better than this. This makes life very simple! When optimizing your images for use in PowerPoint, scale them no larger than your display setting.

PowerPoint resolution

PowerPoint defaults to a resolution of 720 × 540 (approximately the same as digital video). In PowerPoint, select File > Page Setup and you'll see the page is set to 10 × 7.5 inches (25.4 × 19.05 cm). The problem with this dimension is that PowerPoint will scale your presentation visuals either up or down, depending on your current display setting (see above).

So how do you fix this? Using 1024 × 768 for this example, divide each dimension by 72 ppi (pixels per inch). 1024 divided by 72 = 14.22 inches (36.19 cm). Enter this for page width. 768 divided by 72 = 10.66 inches (27.08 cm). Enter this for page height. Your PowerPoint file is now perfectly set for a 1024 × 768 display (Fig. 4.4).

Figure 4.4
Page set up for different display settings.

800x600 11.11" x 8.33" or 28.22cm x 21.16cm
1024x768 14.22" x 10.66" or 36.19cm x 27.08cm
1152x864 16.00" x 12.00" or 40.64cm x 30.48cm

!!!!!!!!!!!!!!!!! Note !

You can save these settings, and every time you open PowerPoint, the blank template will already be formatted for your display. Select File > Save As, choose 'Design Template' as the file type, and type 'Blank' as the filename (the .pot extension will be added automatically). Try it out: select File > Close, then File > New, choose 'Blank' as the template. Select File > Page Setup and note that your page setup has been updated.

Why should you change the page setup? If you keep the default setup, PowerPoint will automatically stretch the slide show to fit your display settings. The difference may not be apparent with every show. However, when image quality is very important to your presentation, and you have spent time resizing and optimizing your images to fit your display, then you should change the page setup.

Printer resolution

The number of pixels (or dots) across a line (the width) of your printed image describes the printer resolution. This is determined by the quality, or settings, of your printer and is a form of output resolution. You can calculate what printed image size you can safely achieve from the dimensions of the original image. A 3000 × 2000-pixel image from a 6-megapixel camera printed at 300 dpi will be 10 inches across the horizontal axis (3000 divided by 300).

Looking at this from another viewpoint, a 1500 × 1000 pixel image printed at a size of 10 inches will be printing at a resolution of 150 dpi (1500 divided by 10). You don't need to remember this but you do need to understand it (Fig. 4.5).

Figure 4.5
Calculating print sizes.

$$\frac{3{,}000 \text{ pixels} \div 300 \text{ dpi}}{10" \text{ print width}}$$

$$\frac{1{,}500 \text{ pixels} \div 10" \text{ print width}}{150 \text{ dpi}}$$

If you are going to print your images you will need to know the resolution of your printer. Clearly, printing an image that resolves to 600 dpi on a 300 dpi printer is just a waste of disk space; you may as well save it at a resolution of 300 dpi. Remember from Chapter 2 that we recommend saving your original image as a master file at the highest resolution available; you might buy a new printer!

Increasing image size

There might be an occasion when you want to increase rather than decrease the dimensions of an image, possibly to make a large poster or to use an image from the web in a presentation. If you just drag the corner of the image to increase its size, or even increase the dimensions using Photoshop Elements, it will pixilate. This might not matter if the image is to be viewed at a distance, but there is a better way to achieve optimum results.

The reason that the image pixilates is that there are gaps between pixels as they are stretched apart. You can use Photoshop Elements to fill those gaps in with color. But, as explained in Chapter 3, this can result in a blurred image. The result will never be as good as an original high-resolution image but it can be adequate for most tasks.

Photoshop can best-guess what color each pixel needs to be. Using Photoshop Elements, open 'lowresolution.jpg' from the Chapter 4 folder on the CD (Fig. 4.6 top left). This is a small image, suitable for use on a website, but we want to enlarge it to use on a poster. You might want to try enlarging it just by increasing the image width to 10 inches by adjusting the image width using Image > Resize > Image size (make sure you choose inches for the scale and that the image is not resampled by unticking the box at the bottom). To see the entire image select View > Fit on screen. The result is pretty disappointing. Now try 'interpolating' the image, by which we mean resizing and getting Photoshop to fill in the gaps between pixels.

Figure 4.6
Top left, low resolution image;
top right, nearest neighbor
resampling; bottom left, bilinear
resampling; bottom right,
bicubic resampling (based on a
photograph by Royal College of
Surgeons Photographic Studios).

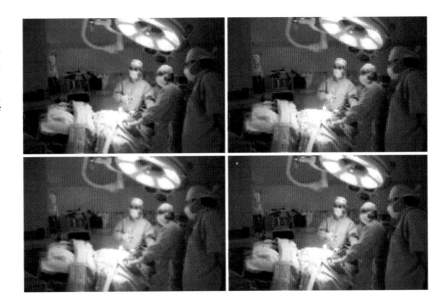

Open the image size dialogue box again (Image > Resize > Image size).
After changing the image width to 6 inches, tick the box at the bottom
labeled 'Resample Image'. You now have three choices. These are the three
methods of interpolation used by Photoshop: 'Nearest Neighbor', 'Bilinear',
and 'Bicubic'. 'Nearest Neighbor' does what the name suggests; it chooses a
color the same as the nearest pixel (Fig. 4.6 top right). 'Bilinear' chooses a
color between neighboring pixels, creating a smoother effect (Fig. 4.6 bottom
left). 'Bicubic' is what we want (Fig. 4.6 bottom right). This is the slowest
technique, as it will select a color based on an average of the nearest 16
pixels. Select 'Bicubic' and click 'OK'. The image is now bigger but does not
pixilate as much. If it looks a little soft, you can sharpen it by selecting
Filter > Sharpen > Unsharp mask. This increases the sharpness of any
image, but beware, only use this once on each image and use it after all other
changes have been made.

!!!!!!!!!!!!!!!!!! Note !   A word of caution regarding interpolation: you can increase image sizes by
any amount that you want but image quality deteriorates the more you try
to do this and it is unwise to increase by much more than 150%.

It is always best to try to anticipate and prevent such problems. One of
the most common images that you might want to enlarge might be a 35 mm
slide. When scanning slides, use as high a resolution as you can, even the
highest available on your scanner. Enlarge the image to the size that you need
and then compress it and save it as a .jpeg.

Conclusion   The issue of resolution is important but simple!
When you save your master image always save it at the highest resolution
available, without enlarging it. When subsequently using images, think of the
output resolution. For presentations or websites, save copies of the image at

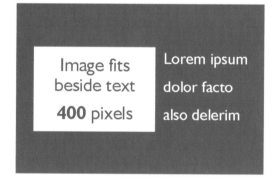

screen resolution (approximately 800 to 1024 pixels wide). For printing
purposes, save at the resolution of your printer (typically 300 or 600 dpi).
    In PowerPoint, an 800-pixel-wide image will fill the screen (if your display
is set for 800 × 600 pixels). If you want to use a title above the image on
your slide, choose approximately 600 pixels wide. If you are going to place
the image beside some text, choose 200–400 pixels for the width (Fig. 4.7).

Chapter 5

PowerPoint® for beginners

Terry Irwin and Julie Terberg

Although PowerPoint® is the world's most popular presentation program, and most medical presenters use it, many people feel intimidated by the program and prefer to give presentations prepared for them by employees or trainees. If you are a complete PowerPoint novice, this chapter is for you. By the time you have read the chapter and completed the tutorials, you will be able to open the program, set up a presentation, choose a template, prepare the presentation and save it in a number of different ways. We will not deal with adding images and video because there is a chapter specifically devoted to this.

To begin with, let's make it easy for you to open PowerPoint whenever you come to use it. We will assume that you are using Windows® XP. If your PowerPoint icon is not easily found, you might want to place it on the Taskbar, in the Start Menu or on your desktop.

To place the icon in the Start Menu click Start > All Programs and look for, but do not click on, the name 'Microsoft PowerPoint'. Click and hold down the mouse button and drag the icon and name of the program to the left until it lies just below the name given to your computer, up above the Start button. As you drag the icon to the correct position a black line will appear (Fig. 5.1). Release the mouse button when you are happy with the position of the icon and it will appear there (Fig. 5.2).

Alternatively, to place the icon on the Taskbar, again find the PowerPoint program icon and program name, and drag it to the Taskbar at the bottom left-hand corner of your desktop, immediately to the right of the Start button. Once again a dark line will appear, but this one is like a capital 'I' (Fig. 5.3).

To place the shortcut on your desktop, minimize all windows that are open. Right-click on the icon in the Taskbar, drag it to the desktop and drop

Figure 5.1
Placing the PowerPoint icon in the Start menu.

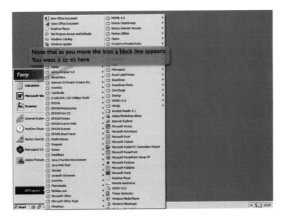

it there. A dialogue box will ask you whether you want to move the icon there or copy it. Choose 'Copy Here'.

Now you can start PowerPoint by clicking either of these icons. Click one now to open the program.

You will be presented with a blank PowerPoint slide. (Fig. 5.4). You might be able to see the task pane to the right of your presentation. If not, click

Figure 5.2
The icon in position in the Start menu.

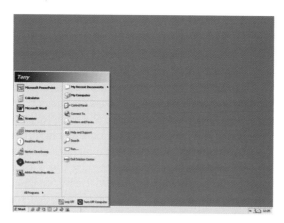

Figure 5.3
Placing the PowerPoint icon in the task bar.

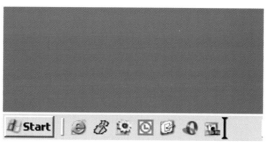

Figure 5.4
Your first slide ready for content.

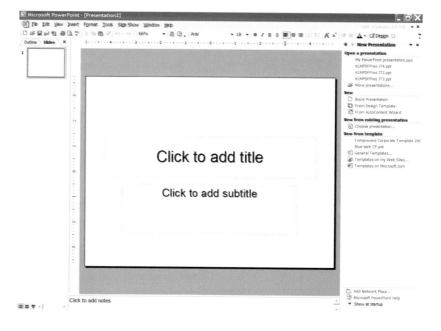

View > Task Pane and it will appear. The task pane lists, from top to bottom: presentations that you have opened recently, options for preparing a new presentation from a blank canvas, an existing template or from a Wizard.

We would not recommend the Wizard, but by all means try it out and form your own opinion. Below these are options to base a presentation on an existing presentation (in reality all this does is use the File > Open command). Last of the choices is the option to open a recently used template. Of course, if you have just installed PowerPoint you will not have any existing presentations or recent templates to work from, so these options will be empty.

Let's look under 'New from template' and then select 'General Templates' in the choices listed above. You will note that the appearance of the task pane now changes to offer up all the design templates installed on your computer. The basic PowerPoint templates will have to do for now! As you read on in the book, we will teach you how to make your own template very easily.

Select any template and click on it. The template is now applied to your slide. In addition, the layout of your slide is automatically set to a title slide. Add a title, say, 'My PowerPoint presentation', and add your name (Fig. 5.5). Now save the presentation (File > Save As) and add a name that is easy to remember.

!!!!!!!!!!!!!!!!!! *Tip:*   Save all your PowerPoint presentations in one place on your computer. You might want to add a folder to your desktop, called 'Presentations', and always save to this. That way they are easy to find.

Note that this name is now displayed along the top of the PowerPoint window, rather than 'Presentation 1'. Get into the habit of saving your files regularly – even as often as every slide that you add.

You might not particularly like the color scheme that is used in the template. You can easily change this. Click the small down-arrow, beside the words 'Slide Layout' at the top right corner of the window. Choose the option Slide Design > Color Schemes. Click on each of the color schemes

Figure 5.5
The title slide.

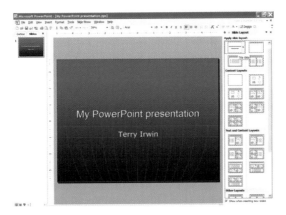

and choose the one you want. Later on you will learn how to choose a color combination that suits the room in which you are presenting. You can always go back to the templates by following the same step and selecting Slide Design > Slide Templates. This option lets you see a visual image of each template available on your computer.

You are ready to add more slides but before you do there is one more important task. You have to determine how you will be presenting your slides.

Select File > Page Setup. You can choose to show your presentation on a multimedia projector or on your computer (On-screen Show), on various sizes of paper (say A4 for printing on to acetates/transparencies) or as 35 mm slides, to be developed by a photographic department or shop. For now choose 'On-screen Show'. Now save again.

Click on the down arrow beside 'Slide Design' and choose 'Slide Layout'.

To add a new slide you can use a number of methods. The easiest is to type 'Ctrl M'. You can use Insert > New Slide or click the button 'New Slide'. On the new slide, click on the 'Title' area and add a title such as 'My second slide'. Now click on the wording 'Click to add text' and put some additional text as bullet points. Note that the bullet points are all towards the top of the slide. Don't be tempted to move this yet – we will teach you the best way to change this later.

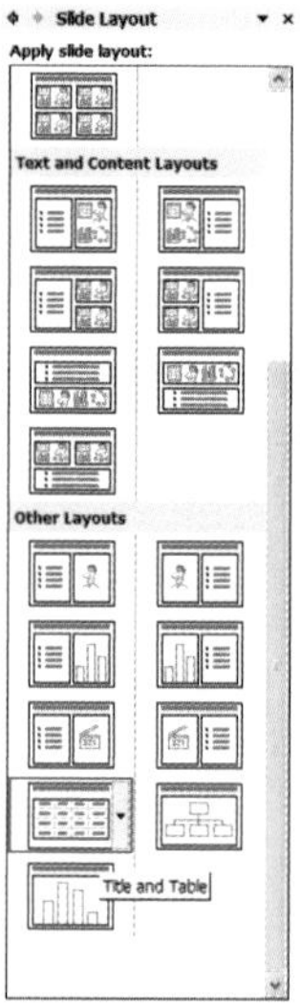

You might find that even if you use a lower-case letter for the start of the first word on each line, PowerPoint changes this to upper case. Many people find it preferable to use lower case. If so, you need to change the default settings. This is easy to do. Select Tools > Autocorrect Options. A dialogue box appears. Remove the tick from the option 'Capitalize first letter of sentences'. You might also want to remove the tick against the option 'Capitalize first letter of table cells'. Click 'OK'. If you add new bullet points in lower case, now the first letter will not automatically be capitalized.

Note that a dotted line surrounds the text box. If you click outside this box it will disappear. If at any time you make a mistake, you can go back by typing 'Ctrl Z' or click the little back arrow on the top menu bar. In Chapter 16 you will learn how to choose the best font and font sizes and how to change these in the slide template, for now, just accept the defaults.

Save your slide (type 'Ctrl S'). Get in the habit of doing this; we will not remind you again!

Next we will add a slide with a table. Type 'Ctrl M' to insert a new slide. In 'Slide Layout', scroll down until you see the 'Other layouts' and click the one that shows a title and table (Fig. 5.6).

Give your slide the title 'Table'. Now double-click to add a table, where indicated. Choose two columns and eight rows. Add some data to the table as shown in Figure 5.7. Don't worry about formatting the table yet.

Next, open a new slide ('Ctrl M') and choose the layout for a chart. Give your slide a title such as 'Chart'. Double-click where indicated to insert a chart. A chart and data table appears. Place the cursor over the top left gray box and hit the 'Delete' key to remove all the data.

Now add the data shown in Figure 5.8. Note that the graph builds as you add the data. We have increased the size of the first data box to let you see all of the text. The legend 'No. of patients' is distracting set off to the right.

Figure 5.6   The Slide Layout menu.

Figure 5.7
Inserting a table.

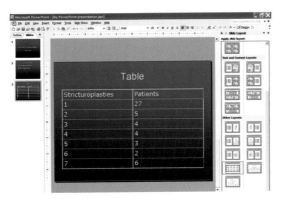

Figure 5.8
Inserting a graph.

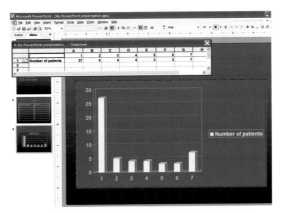

Make sure that the data table is still visible (if not double-click on the graph) and then click on the legend. Right-click on it and select 'Format Legend' and then the 'Placement' tab. Choose 'Top'. This is preferable to dragging the legend to this position because PowerPoint resizes the graph at the same time as moving the legend. If you don't want a label at all, select the legend and delete it.

Now let's change the color of the graph. Make sure that the drawing menu is visible. If you cannot see it, then right-click with the cursor over the top gray menu bar and make sure that 'Drawing' is ticked (Fig. 5.9). Click on any of the vertical bars in the chart. All of the bars will be highlighted (note the small square at the corners). Click on the small down-arrow beside the fill color icon and choose a different color (Fig. 5.10). Another way to achieve the same effect is to click on the legend, then click on the colored box next to the legend to highlight it, and then choose a fill color as above.

You can format the wall of the chart area by right-clicking on the chart anywhere that is blank and selecting 'Format walls'. Select a different color and see how it works. In general it is best to use the default settings if you are new to PowerPoint. You could choose any color you like, or be really adventurous and select 'Fill Effects'. Choose the 'Picture' tab and then select 'Picture'. Choose the image 'Crohns' from the chapter folder on the CD and insert it by clicking 'OK' twice.

Now carefully right-click on one of the horizontal gridlines and choose 'Format Gridlines'. If you get the option 'Format walls', you have missed the

Figure 5.9
Opening the Drawing menu.

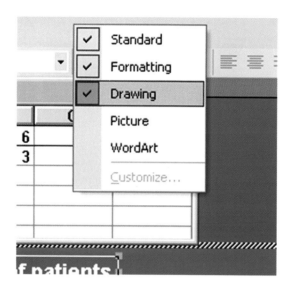

Figure 5.10
Changing the fill colors. Note that each of the columns is highlighted with a small square at each corner.

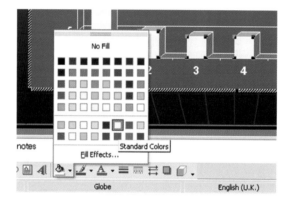

line. Try again! Select the options shown in Figure 5.11. Now hold the cursor over the lower edge of the chart near the numbers, until a pop-up box says 'Category Axis'. Right-click here, choose 'Format Axis' and select a similar blue color for the lines, but leave it solid. Select the 'Font' tab and change the color to a pale blue/gray. Do the same for the vertical axis and for the chart walls (to select this, place the cursor between the vertical axis on the left and the first column, then right-click and select 'Format walls'). Click outside the graph to close the data table.

Your graph should now look like Figure 5.12! Are you saving your presentation?

If you are feeling really adventurous you can animate the graph. You will learn in Chapter 18 that this should not be overdone – less is more! Click the down-arrow to the right of where it says 'Slide Layout' (if the task pane is not visible select View > Task Pane) and choose 'Custom Animation'. Now (single-) click on the graph. Click on Add Effect > Entrance > Wipe. Click the down arrow to the right of 'chart 2' and choose 'Start With Previous' and then click the arrow again and choose 'Effect Options'. Leave the 'Effect' and 'Timing' tabs unchanged. In the 'Chart Animation' tab choose

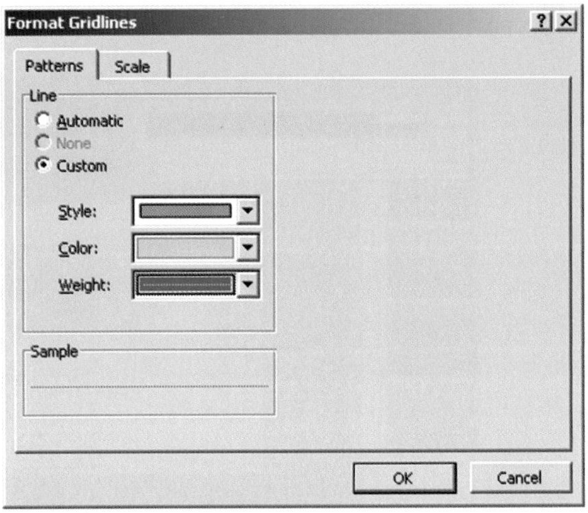

Figure 5.11
Formatting the gridlines.

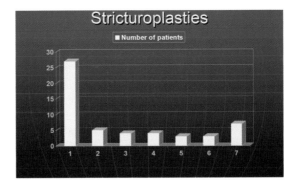

Figure 5.12
The finished graph.

'By element in series' and uncheck the 'Animate grid and legend' box. Click 'OK'.

In the 'Custom Animation' pane to the right of your work space you will now see a double down-arrow below the 'chart 2' series. Click to open the rest of the animation. If you leave these as they are, each column in the graph will build on a mouse click – an effect that can be useful. If you want the chart to build itself, hold the shift key and click on each line that says 'chart 2 series item' in turn, then click the down arrow and select 'Start After Previous'. By default, the timing will be set to 0.5 seconds, but you can change this if you wish by clicking the down arrow again and selecting 'Timing'.

Now you can add a pie chart. Using the data in the chart above, build another identical slide but do not change the chart background color, gridlines or fonts. Now click Chart > Chart Type. Choose 'Pie' and select the center option in the lower row (Fig. 5.13).

The pie chart has no labels so it is hard to work out what each segment means. Click on any of the segments. All the segments should be highlighted. Right-click and select 'Format Data Series'. Now uncheck all of the options in the data labels tab except 'Percentage'. Go to the 'Patterns' tab and select 'None' for the border option. Go to the 'Options' tab and try changing the angle of the first slice to see how you want the pie chart orientated

Figure 5.13
Inserting a pie chart.

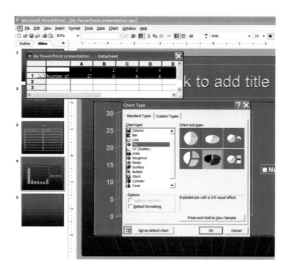

Figure 5.14
The finished pie chart.

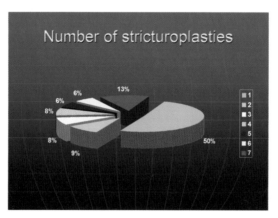

(we choose 20 degrees). OK, we're starting to play now, but that is the best way to learn PowerPoint!

There should be two boxes around your chart. The outer one is the chart area and the inner one is the plot area. If the outer one is not visible double-click anywhere on the chart. This will also bring up the data series. The plot area should be marked by a solid line; if this is not visible, click just to the right of the pie chart. Now place the mouse over the plot area line until a little pop-up box says 'Plot Area' and then right-click and select 'Format Plot Area' to make changes to this portion of your chart. In particular, you might want to remove the line around it by choosing 'None' for the 'Border' option. You should now have a slide that looks like Figure 5.14.

Now we will add a Venn diagram. PowerPoint can do this very easily. Type 'Ctrl M' to add a new slide. Choose either the slide layout that has a title only or open any slide layout and delete the body by clicking on it and hitting the 'Delete' key. Select Insert > Diagram and choose a 'Venn diagram' from the options (middle option on lower row; see Fig. 5.15). Give the slide the title 'Who cares'. Click over each of the three labels and add the words 'carers', 'primary physician', and 'secondary physician'. You might want a

Figure 5.15
Inserting a Venn diagram.

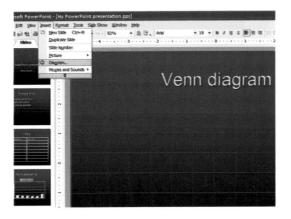

Figure 5.16
A finished Venn diagram.

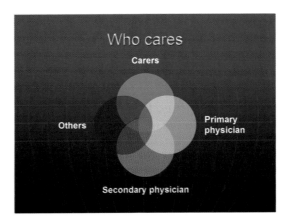

fourth category. To add another circle, right-click on any of the circles and choose 'Insert shape'. Type the word 'others' against this shape. You can resize the diagram by selecting Layout > Expand Diagram from the diagram toolbar that should be floating on your slide. Drag the corners to change size, click on the outer box and hold the mouse down to move the whole diagram. Now click the 'AutoFormat' button on the diagram toolbar (this is the button between 'Layout' and 'Change to'). If it suits your needs, you can now change the appearance of the diagram. Your final diagram might look like Figure 5.16. Transparency is not supported in PowerPoint versions earlier than Office XP (PowerPoint 2002) so you might get a stippled fill rather than that seen in the figure.

A Venn diagram is not always suitable for every occasion. Try the 'Change to' option and select each diagram type in turn. You can see that there are plenty of variations – enough to suit most needs.

You might like to try this variation. Right-click on one of the circles and select 'Delete shape'. Once again, right-click on a circle in the Venn diagram and select 'Format AutoShape'. Now click the down arrow next to 'Color' and choose 'Fill Effects', the 'Picture' tab, and then 'Select Picture'. Choose 'surgeon' from the chapter folder. Click 'OK' twice. Repeat this for the other circles, selecting the images 'nurse' and 'anesthesiology'. Label each circle

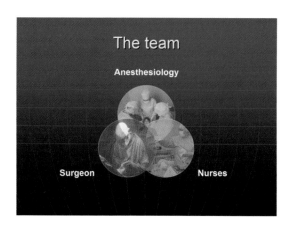

Figure 5.17
An alternative Venn diagram
with images filling the circles.

with the corresponding image names. Give the slide the title 'The team'. You
should have a Venn diagram that looks like Figure 5.17.

Have you been saving your presentation? Imagine if you lost all this work!
Our completed presentation is saved in the chapter folder as 'My PowerPoint
presentation'.

Now you can go back to the first slide either by choosing it in the 'Slides'
tab to the left or by scrolling up to it. Click on the 'Slide Show' icon in the
bottom left corner or simply hit the 'F5' key. You can advance slides using the
left mouse button, the 'Enter' key or the right arrow key.

Later in the book you will learn how to give an effective presentation. For
now, especially as you practice, you might want to use 'Speaker Notes'. To do
so, select View > Notes Page. For each slide, type in some reminders of
what you want to say. You can go from slide to slide in 'Notes' view by using
the scroll bar to the right.

As your first slide appears in Slideshow mode, right-click on the slide and
select 'Speaker Notes'. Then advance the slides in the usual way. With each
slide you will see your own notes. Try this with the presentation saved in the
chapter folder.

You might find that you are giving a talk using acetates and an overhead
projector. This style of presentation is getting much less common but it is
cheap and cheerful, and still has its place. It might be a necessary evil because
the venue where you are presenting does not lend itself to data projection,
or the meeting might be of a type that just does not justify lugging a
projector from the car to the room in a downpour!

To create a presentation suitable for acetates you need to start again!

Open PowerPoint as before. Select File > Page Setup and from the
'Slides sized for:' drop-down menu, choose the size of acetate that you are
using (say A4). Usually it is easier to select 'Portrait' mode rather than
'Landscape', but that is a matter of personal opinion.

Do not choose a template, just type straight in to the title area and add
your name as before. Now add a new slide (Ctrl M) and then select
View > Master > Slide Master. Delete the 'Date' and 'Number' areas. In
the 'Footer' area, type 'this side towards screen'. Now each of your slides
will have that text at the bottom, but it will be out of sight and the audience
will not see it. That way, you will always know which direction to face the

Figure 5.18
A basic template for overhead projection.

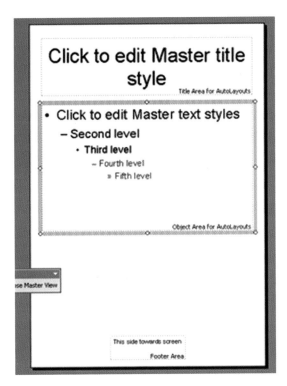

acetate! No more turning it over eight times to get it right. Now you want to set up the area into which you will type. Most overhead projectors have a square glass area. You want to drag the bottom of the text area up until the viewable area of the slide is roughly square (Fig. 5.18). Select 'Close Master View'.

You can now add slides in exactly the same way as you learned for on-screen presentation. Remember that there is no point adding animation! You can create your acetates in color but this will be expensive if you are printing a lot of acetates. However, for an important presentation it might be worth considering.

In these exercises you have created a PowerPoint presentation containing a title slide, bullet points, a table, a graph and a diagram. Now that you have mastered the basics, in the next chapters we will teach you how to design your own background templates, and how to add images and video.

Before we finish, you need to know how to save your presentation ready to show it. So far, you have just saved the file, but as what? If you select File > Save As, you will see that by default you saved it as a type called 'Presentation'. This means that you can go back to it and modify it. If you are happy that the presentation is finished, you might choose to save it as a 'PowerPoint Show', which has the suffix '.pps' rather than '.ppt.' This means that when you open the file it will open in 'Slide Show' mode, with the first slide open and ready to show to your audience. This saves all that hunting around for the show icon! The .pps file can be edited in PowerPoint, although you will need to open PowerPoint first, and then open the .pps file – it will not launch the program automatically like a .ppt file will.

Figure 5.19
The package for CD option
in PowerPoint 2003.

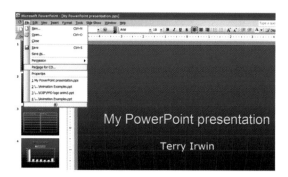

You can save the presentation for the web, but more of that in Chapter 8. You might also choose to save it in an older version of PowerPoint. This is useful if you are showing it on a computer that only has a previous version of PowerPoint, because it may not recognize your presentation otherwise. If in doubt, always check before you take your talk on the road, or bring several versions.

PowerPoint 2003 has a neat option called 'Package for CD', which allows you to prepare a presentation on a CD using a 'Wizard' (Fig. 5.19). It adds all of the necessary files, including video files (which, as you will learn in Chapter 6, can cause problems) and also adds an 'Autostart' file so that when you insert the CD into a computer it plays your presentation without prompting. The program even burns the CD. Neat!

Creating a custom PowerPoint® template

Julie Terberg and Terry Irwin

We have all seen presentations created with standard templates and backgrounds. These presentations tend to look basic, boring, and very unoriginal. It is not that difficult to use your imagination to create a unique background more suited to your presentation topic. By following a few simple steps to customizing your slide masters, you are on your way to a creative and effective presentation.

Your CD includes 20 custom-designed templates (they are free for you to use; however, you must not give them away, sell them, or post them on the web). You might want to take a look at the way these templates are formatted before you begin your custom design. We have used PowerPoint® 2002 to create the templates in this chapter. When the commands are drastically different, we will explain how to accomplish them using older versions of PowerPoint.

Determine final presentation environment

Before you begin designing a new template, you need to consider how your presentation is going to be viewed. Will it be projected to a large or small audience? Will it be delivered on a laptop to a handful of people around a conference table? Will you be converting your presentation to .html and delivering it on the internet? Will there be a lot of light in the room or will you be in front of a lighted podium in a darkened room?

If your presentation environment will be brightly lit, your visuals will be easier to read on a white or light background with dark text. If the room will be dark, use a medium to dark background with white or light text. In a dark environment, a white screen will glow, making it uncomfortable to read from. And, if you are creating a web-based presentation, it is best to stick with a light to medium background with black or dark-colored text.

Only using handouts? Keep your backgrounds primarily white and use full-color for accents, photos, and graphics.

Gather existing materials

If your hospital, group, or company has a public relations or marketing department then you should visit it first. One of the objectives of such a department is to develop standards for print and other media, maintaining some consistency with logos, typography, and images. There will probably be digital files of approved logos and images that you can use. Ask if there is a standard template that you should use for your presentation, or if there are guidelines for you to follow. If you are not enthusiastic about the material the department wants you to work from, buy them a copy of this book!

Chances are, if you are reading this chapter then you are on your own for the template design. Before you design anything, gather all of the elements you already have to put into your presentation: logos, graphics, charts, photos or digital images, and an outline or script of your presentation. Determine what types of visuals you will be creating: mainly text, some graphics, a few charts, a lot of photographs or a mix of everything? Pull out a good sampling of visuals that you can use when developing your presentation template.

One of those editing decisions that troubled us when we were writing this book was where to position this chapter. If you need to know how to plan your presentation before you design the template, you might want to read Chapter 18 on effective presentations at this stage. It will help you plan your presentation, which will guide how to build your slideshow.

Determine display size

Before you begin designing a template, determine your final presentation display size. What is this? The display size or 'screen area' is the number of pixels that your monitor is currently set to display. The higher the number of pixels, the more information you can display on your screen. The two most common settings (at the time this chapter was written) are 800×600 and 1024×768. Although your monitor might be capable of displaying a higher resolution, if you are going to share your presentation with others you will want to stick with either of these settings. If you are using a projector, you will need to check the manual for the maximum projector display setting. If necessary, change the settings on your monitor or laptop to match the projector. If you are unsure of the setting, select 800×600.

Windows® *users*: to check your current display setting, use the right mouse button on your desktop (right-click) and then select 'Properties' or click Start > Settings > Control Panel, and double-click the 'Display' icon. In the 'Display Properties' dialogue box, select the 'Settings' tab. In the lower right corner is the 'Screen area'; these pixel dimensions indicate your current settings. You can slide the arrow up or down to the next setting if necessary; click 'Apply' to reset your display (Fig. 6.1).

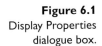

Figure 6.1
Display Properties
dialogue box.

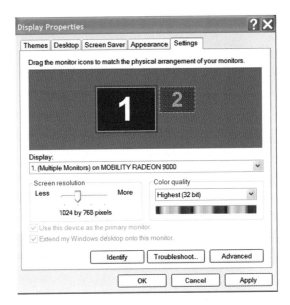

Develop background images

You have unlimited design options when creating a new background for your presentation. Take a look at the examples included on the CD for design inspiration. Backgrounds come in many different graphic varieties but we will focus on two main types: abstract and photographic.

Abstract backgrounds

An abstract background is non-descriptive and can be useful for a variety of topics. Abstracts are fairly simple to construct in Photoshop Elements®. Starting with just about any digital image, you can apply filters, merge layers, and colorize the final abstract.

To follow the first example, in Photoshop Elements, open the file 'Blur original.tif' from the Chapter 6 folder on the CD. It looks like a nice medical image – but not for long, as soon it will be an abstract background.

Select File > Save As, change the filename to 'Abstract1' (or whatever you like) choose Photoshop (.psd) as the format, and click 'Save'. And now have some fun! From the top menu bar, select Filter > Blur > Motion Blur, change the angle to 15° and the distance to 450 pixels (Fig. 6.2).

The next step in making this abstract work as a background is to resize the image. Select Image > Resize > Image Size. In the 'Image Size' dialogue box, uncheck the box for 'Constrain Proportions'. Change the width and height to reflect the pixel dimensions for your presentation display setting (800 × 600 or 1024 × 768) and select 'OK'. Type 'Ctrl S' to save the file.

For this example, let's assume that the presentation environment will not have a lot of ambient light, which means that a darker background will work best (with white or light text for the most contrast and legibility). Our example, 'Abstract1', will need to be darker, have less contrast, and even fewer colors, to work effectively. Type 'Ctrl U', or select Enhance > Adjust Color > Hue/Saturation. Click the 'Colorize' button in the lower right corner. You can adjust the sliders to achieve the hue (color), saturation, and

Figure 6.2
Motion Blur dialogue box.

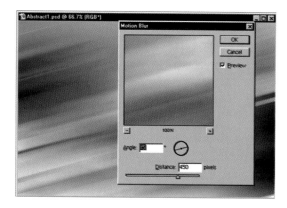

Figure 6.3
Hue/saturation dialogue box.

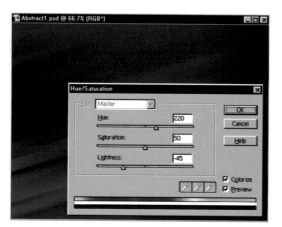

lightness. To achieve the effect shown in this example, use these numbers: hue, 220; saturation, 50; and lightness, −45. The resulting image is a rich blue abstract, perfect for using as a presentation background. Select File > Save As, rename the file 'Abstract Blue' and save as a .jpeg; choose '10' for the image quality when prompted (Fig. 6.3).

Another way to adjust colors in Photoshop Elements is to use the 'Color Variations' tool. Select File > Open Recent and choose 'Abstract1.psd'. Select Enhance > Adjust Color > Color Variations. This dialogue box shows you a preview of multiple color adjustments, all in one window. You can increase or decrease red, green, or blue; darken or lighten your image; adjust the amount of intensity for each adjustment; and make changes to midtones, shadows, highlights, or saturation. Explore these options to learn more about them and how they affect your image. Have a target color range in mind: blues, greens, or whatever suits your presentation best. If you go too far with your variations, just click on the 'Before' image (or click 'Reset Color') to return to the original image colors. Keep in mind that your presentation background should not have a lot of contrast. Tone-down light areas on dark backgrounds, and vice versa (Fig. 6.4).

Try other filters to create different abstract effects. Combine filters and color adjustments for the most variety. These four abstract examples all began from the same file: 'blur original.tif' (Fig. 6.5).

Figure 6.4
Color Variations dialogue box.

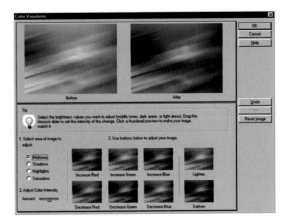

Figure 6.5
All of these templates were
produced from the blur
original.tif.

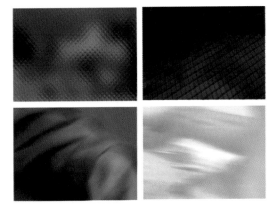

Photographic backgrounds

As the name implies, photographic backgrounds are made up of digital photos or images. They are descriptive and should coordinate with your presentation topic. Some backgrounds consist of one large, subdued image; others might be a montage of multiple images, and still others might have objects or people clipped out of their original image and artfully ghosted on another background. You can create an abstract background and then place a series of small photos along one edge, and so on. The combinations are almost unlimited.

When selecting a photograph to use for a background image, the subject matter should be your first consideration (it should complement your presentation topic!). Next, you will need an image large enough for your display size, or a larger image that you can crop. If you try to resize your image larger, it may become pixilated (see Chapter 4). You should also look for a rather simple image; try not to have too much going on in the background. Remember, the information should be the focus of your presentation, not the background.

To follow along with the first photographic background example, open the file 'Hands original.tif' from the Chapter 6 folder on the CD.

Select the 'Eye-dropper tool', hold down the 'Alt' key and select a dark blue pixel from the top left. This will change the background color to a dark blue.

Select File > New ('Ctrl N'). Name the file 'Photo hands', set the width to '800 pixels', the height to '600 pixels', resolution to '72', the mode to 'RGB', and the contents to 'Background color' (Fig. 6.6).

Click on the 'Hands original.tif' window and type 'Ctrl A' to select the entire image and then 'Ctrl C' to copy it. Switch back to the new blue file and type 'Ctrl V' to paste the hands photo. Click and drag the image to move it up and over slightly to the left, so that the hands are visible on the right side of the window. Select Image > Resize > Scale, and in the properties toolbar at the top, click the chain icon to maintain aspect ratio and type '85%' in one of the dimensions. Reposition the image so that it is snug to the top of the window.

Next, in the layers window, select 'Layer 1', and change the opacity to '25%' (Fig. 6.7).

Figure 6.6
Settings for the new file.

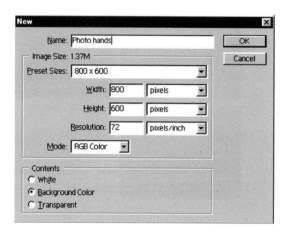

Figure 6.7
Setting the layers window.

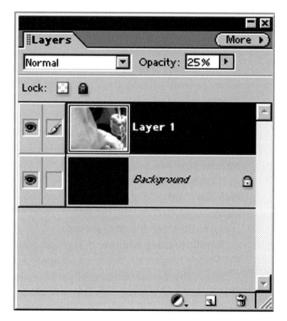

Save as a .jpeg file with a new name. The resulting photographic background is interesting yet not too complex to be a workable presentation background. The focal point (fingers with instrument) has been shifted to the right of the frame, giving you more legibility for type and graphics to be placed on top (Fig. 6.8).

For the next photographic background, open the file 'Abstract Green.jpg' from the chapter folder on the CD. Next, open the file 'Dental.tif' from the same folder. Type 'M' to select the Marquee tool, and click and drag a selection box down the center of the dental image (Fig. 6.9).

Click and drag this selection to the 'Abstract Green.jpg' window to create a new layer (or type 'Ctrl C' to copy, and then switch to the green background and type 'Ctrl V' to paste). Select Image > Resize > Scale, and in the properties toolbar at the top, click the chain icon to maintain aspect ratio, and type '43%' in one of the dimensions. Reposition this layer so that it fits snugly along the right side of the frame.

The next step is to re-color the dental image. Type 'Ctrl U' to bring up the hue/saturation dialogue box. Click the 'Colorize' box and change the hue to

Figure 6.8
Simple photographic background (photography by Royal College of Surgeons Photographic Studios).

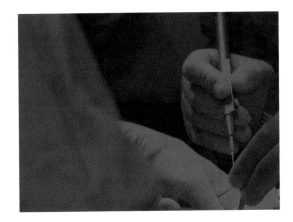

Figure 6.9
Marquee selection (photography by Royal College of Surgeons Photographic Studios).

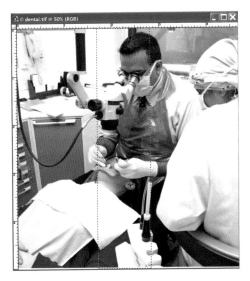

Figure 6.10
Abstract and photographic
background combined
(photography by Royal College
of Surgeons Photographic
Studios).

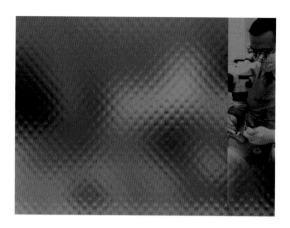

Figure 6.11
An appropriate background can
enhance your presentation.

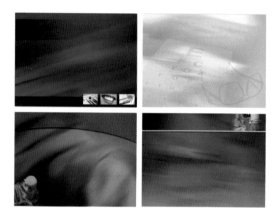

'160,' saturation to '20,' and lightness to '−50'. Click 'OK' to apply. Select File > Save As and save your file as a .jpeg with a new file name.

Now let's give the bottom edge of the photo a soft edge to blend it into the abstract background. Type 'M' to select the Marquee selection tool, and click and drag a selection rectangle encompassing about the bottom third of the dental image.

Choose Select from the top menu bar, then 'Feather' and change the feather radius to 15 pixels. Click 'OK'. Type 'Ctrl X' (or Edit > Cut) to omit the selected area. Remember to save your file (Fig. 6.10).

Photographic backgrounds can enhance your presentation and reinforce your topic or message. Remember to stick with simple images, subdue the color palette, and move the main focal point away from the central portion of the screen. Add simple graphics like rectangles and lines to enhance your background, and create an area for titles or other text elements. A few more photographic backgrounds for inspiration are shown in Figure 6.11.

Format PowerPoint slide masters

Now that you have created a custom background, it's time to use it to develop your presentation masters. Open PowerPoint and begin with a new blank presentation. Select View > Master > Slide Master.

Figure 6.12
Default text placeholders.

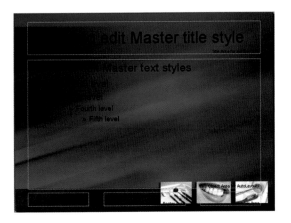

! ! ! ! ! ! ! ! ! ! ! ! ! ! ! ! ! ! *Note !* PowerPoint 2002 defaults to Arial text; older versions default to Times New Roman.

Select Format > Background, click the small, black drop-down arrow, select 'Fill Effects' and then the 'Picture' tab. Click 'Select Picture' and then navigate to the Chapter 6 folder on the CD. Select the file 'Abstract Dental.jpg', 'Insert', and 'OK'. Select File > Save, select the 'Save as type: Design Template' and give your template a name such as 'Blue Dental'.

Let's keep this slide master uncluttered for now, and delete the three placeholders along the bottom: 'date/time, footer, and number area' (Fig. 6.12).

! ! ! ! ! ! ! ! ! ! ! ! ! ! ! ! ! *Note !* You can add any of them back in later by selecting Format > Master Layout and choosing which placeholders to include.

Edit color scheme

You should have noticed right away that the black text will not work with this background. The best way to correct this is by editing the color palette, and establishing the colors to be used for this template. Select Format > Slide Design, choose 'Color Schemes' from the top of the task pane and then 'Edit Color Schemes' near the bottom (Fig. 6.13). (For older versions of PowerPoint: select Format > Slide Color Scheme, then 'Custom'.)

In the Edit Color Schemes dialogue box, select the 'Custom' tab (if not automatically directed). Change each of the scheme colors to better complement your chosen background; remember contrast and legibility are most important. For the Blue Dental example, the background color should be dark blue, text and lines should be white, shadows dark blue, and title text white or very light blue.

You should also edit the next four color swatches to use throughout your presentation. These four colors will remain on the top row of your color palette and you can choose them for filling shapes or using as accent colors. Any charts that you create will be automatically formatted using these colors first. When you are finished editing, choose 'Apply' (Fig. 6.14).

Figure 6.13
Microsoft Office task pane,
PowerPoint 2002.

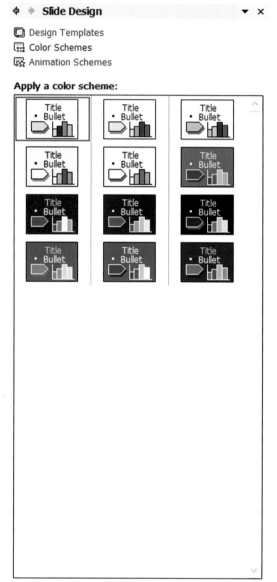

Edit Color Schemes...

!!!!!!!!!!!!!!!!!!! *Note !*   You can return here for further editing as you develop more of your sample slides; you can also tweak the colors if necessary.

Almost all of the standard colors are all highly saturated (very vivid) (Fig. 6.15). If you desire less saturated colors (more subtle,) select the Custom tab from the top of the Background dialogue box, and choose a color from the lower half of the color palette (Fig. 6.16). Type 'Ctrl S' to save your changes.

Figure 6.14
Edit color scheme
dialogue box.

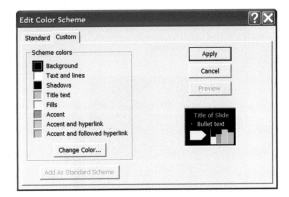

Figure 6.15
Standard colors.

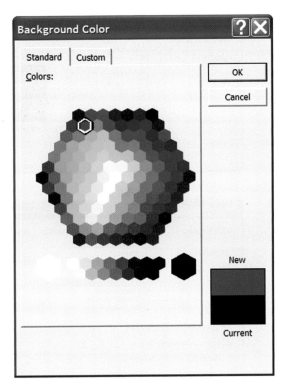

Snap to grid

Type 'Ctrl G' (or select View > Grid and Guides), select 'Snap Objects to Grid', and click 'OK'. Using the Snap to Grid tool allows you to line up text and objects much quicker and helps you achieve a much cleaner and professional presentation. (In older versions of PowerPoint, select Draw > Snap > To Grid from the lower left toolbar.)

Format text placeholders

Next, we need to format the text placeholders and correct their position on the screen. Select the Title Area and change the font to Verdana (users of older versions of PowerPoint can use Arial). In the toolbar at the top of your work area, change the size to 38 and the Alignment to Left ('Ctrl L'). Next, select

Figure 6.16
Custom colors.

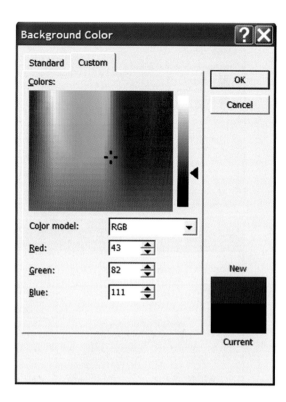

Figure 6.17
Format text dialogue box.

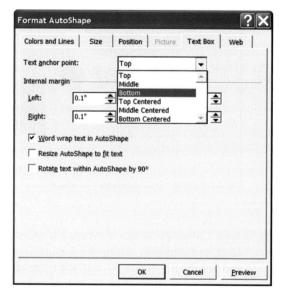

Format > Placeholder, choose the 'Text Box' tab, change the Text Anchor Point to 'Bottom', and click 'OK'. Resetting this text anchor point to the bottom establishes the base point for your titles and allows any two-line titles to wrap up to the top line. Plus, the spacing from your baseline to the body text will always remain the same. It might seem like a small point to make but it really will improve the consistency in your presentation (Fig. 6.17).

With your Title Area still selected, click Format > Line Spacing, change the Line Spacing to 0.9 lines, and click 'OK'. Now select the Object Area (Text Placeholder) and choose Format > Line Spacing again. Change Line Spacing to 0.9 lines, and Before Paragraph to 0.55 lines. By editing the Line Spacing to a slightly smaller amount, and increasing the spacing between paragraphs (or bullet points), you will make your text easier to read.

Bullet points

Place your cursor on the top line of bulleted text and select Format > Bullets and Numbering. Choose the square bullet points at the top right and change the color to one of the accents (the example uses orange). The square bullets are a better complement to the right angles in this particular background image. The second level bullets default to an 'en dash'. Leave this alone – the en dash works well to separate your second-level text from the main bullet points. You should not have to format the last three levels; your text should never be so complicated that you need three levels of bullets. In the rare event that you do need them, the third and fifth levels should be the same bullet type as your first level; the fourth should remain an en dash.

! ! ! ! ! ! ! ! ! ! ! ! ! ! ! ! ! Note !

You have the option to select a picture bullet and to customize your bullet points with a symbol. Use these options carefully and keep your bullet points simple. Complicated bullet points are distracting. Remember to save your changes ('Ctrl S').

The next thing you need to do with this slide master is to reposition the placeholders. Type 'Ctrl A' to select all, or hold down the Shift key and select both placeholders. Hit the down-arrow key on your keyboard six times, or drag the placeholders down. The objective here is to have the Title Area placeholder sitting comfortably within the darker area at the top and the Text Area placeholder a bit underneath this dark area. You can select the handle at the bottom of the Text Area placeholder and move it up above the three images.

Inserting a logo

You have the option of designing your backgrounds in Photoshop with any logos merged to the background image. The problem with this arises when printing your presentation for handouts – the background image and logos will both drop out. A much better solution is to add the logo to the Slide and Title Masters in PowerPoint. This will also allow you to reuse the background for different presentations.

If you want your logo to 'float' on the background it will need a transparent background. If you do not have access to this type of file, you can attempt to edit the file you do have. Review Chapter 3, and specifically the section on Transparency, for details on how to save your logo as a .png file with a transparent background in Photoshop Elements.

Select Insert > Picture > From File and choose 'Smith Logo Drop.png' from the Chapter 6 folder. Drag this logo down to the lower left, aligning it with the left edge of the placeholders. If you choose to, you can scale down the size of the logo slightly. Type 'Ctrl S' to save your template (Fig. 6.18).

Figure 6.18
Slide master with logo in place.

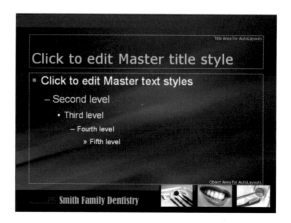

Figure 6.19
Title master with logo in place.

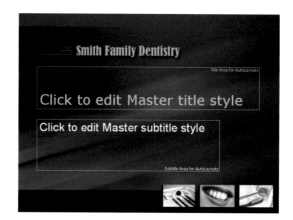

Title Master

Your presentation will need to have a title slide, an introduction, and maybe even a few section headings. These types of slides are formatted using a title master. When developing your presentation background, consider ways you could change the graphics slightly to distinguish your title slides from the main presentation. You can achieve this by increasing the size of your title area, moving any graphics or lines towards the center of the image, and so on. Take a look at the templates on the CD for more ideas.

Select Insert > New Title Master. Your new title master will be formatted with the same font, colors and background image as the slide master.

Select Format > Background > Fill Effects > Picture > Select Picture, then from the chapter folder on the CD select 'Abstract Dental Title.jpg' and click 'OK'. Notice how the dark blue fade in the background has been made larger. Move the Title Area placeholder up, so that it is just above horizontal center. Select the Subtitle Area placeholder, change the alignment to left ('Ctrl L'), and move it to the left to line up with the Title Area.

You can further distinguish the title slides from the rest of the presentation by moving the logo up above the title placeholder, and making it a little larger (Fig. 6.19).

Type 'Ctrl S' to save your changes, and close the file.

Figure 6.20
The finished slide set.

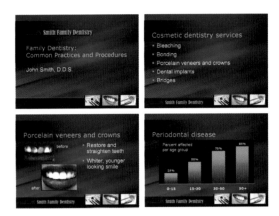

Develop sample slides

Start a new presentation ('Ctrl N' or File > New). Select 'Blue Dental' from the 'Design Templates' in the task pane. If it does not appear automatically in the list, choose 'Browse' from the bottom of the task pane and locate the Blue Dental template. Create a sample slide to represent each type of slide you will be using in your presentation. Examples might include: a title slide, a bulleted text slide, a bar chart, a line chart, a photograph with text, and a quote. Save your sample slides as a presentation (Fig. 6.20).

Put your samples to the test

Before developing the rest of your presentation, take the time to project your samples and review them. Match the final presentation set up as closely as possible: check the display settings, same version of PowerPoint, screen size, room size, and lighting. Sit in various positions around the room and make sure that everything is legible and visible. If you don't like a color, a font, the background image, whatever, now is the time to make changes. Can't read smaller text? Make it larger. If you do make revisions, remember to save as a Design template for future presentations.

Chapter 7

Adding images and video to PowerPoint®

Julie Terberg and Terry Irwin

Having read through the introductory chapters, by now you should have a reasonable grasp of what we are going to say in this chapter. We have already dealt with why images should be cropped, sized, and optimized before they are added to PowerPoint® rather than attempting to do this afterwards and in this chapter we are going to fine tune the skills that you have learned so far, using a series of hands-on, practical lessons.

!!!!!!!!!!!!!!!!!! Note !

You can use any version of PowerPoint for this exercise. The examples were created with PowerPoint 2002. We will highlight any important differences from earlier versions.

To follow along with the exercises, start PowerPoint and select File > Open, choose 'Design Templates' from the 'Files of type' drop-down menu, navigate to the 'PowerPoint templates' folder on the CD and open the template 'Blue Grid.pot'. If you prefer, you can work with one of your own template designs.

!!!!!!!!!!!!!!!!!! Note !

The .pot file extension refers to PowerPoint templates; the .ppt file extension refers to PowerPoint presentation files.

The PowerPoint templates included on the companion CD are free for your personal use. Refer to Chapter 22 for more information about how to access them, change them, and save them to your own system for future presentations.

The PowerPoint template 'Blue Grid' has been formatted to include a sample title slide and a text slide, a color palette, and two 'print version' slides. You can leave these slides alone for now.

Inserting a logo

A great majority of presentations will require a logo of some kind to be placed on the opening slide, if not all of the slides. There are so many different kinds of logos, nearly every shape and color imaginable, that it would be impossible to include instructions on formatting each style for use in a presentation. Some corporate affairs or medical photography departments will develop standards for using a logo in a presentation and, whenever possible, you should refer to this information first.

If you are on your own, here are a few rules for the effective use of logos in your presentation. Use contrast to separate the logo from the background image. If you have a dark-colored logo and you need to put it on a dark background, try inverting the colors in Photoshop Elements® ('Ctrl I' or Image > Adjust > Invert). You should definitely avoid placing a dark logo in a white rectangle on top of a dark background (and vice versa: avoid a light-colored logo in a dark rectangle on top of a light background). This is a fairly common mistake and will make your presentation look amateurish (Figs 7.1 and 7.2). Also, you should find and use a good quality logo. Those captured from websites are too low in resolution and will look pixilated in your presentation. Refer to Chapter 3 for instructions on how to get rid of a solid color surrounding a logo and how to save the logo with a transparent background.

Make sure you are on Slide 1 in PowerPoint and select View > Master > Slide Master. Select Insert > Picture > From File and choose 'HCSlogo.png' from the chapter folder.

Figure 7.1
Avoid using logos in rectangles.

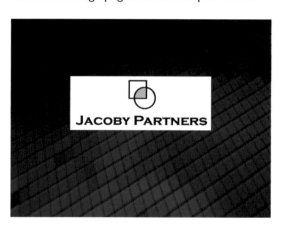

Figure 7.2
Better version of same logo.

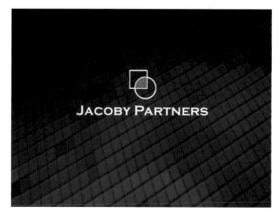

!!!!!!!!!!!!!!!!!! *Note !*   The .png file format supports transparency and true color.

This will place the circular logo in the center of the screen. Hold down the 'Shift' key (to constrain along perpendicular axis) and drag the logo up above the title area. The logo is a bit too large for this layout. Double-click on the logo to bring up the 'Format Picture' dialogue box. Click the 'Size' tab, make sure that 'Lock aspect ratio' is checked, and change the height (or width) dimension to '70%'. The smaller logo will shift to the left, how do you move it back to the exact vertical center?

It is important to line up your logos, text, and images. Whether you choose to align them in relationship to the slide or to each other, there are a couple of ways to establish correct alignment.

Click the Draw button on the lower left menu, then Align or Distribute and select Relative to Slide. Choose Draw > Align or Distribute again, and select Align Center. The HCS logo will move to the vertical center (Fig. 7.3).

The second way to align objects in PowerPoint is to use guides. Type 'Ctrl G' (or select View > Grid and Guides) to bring up the 'Grid and Guides' dialogue box. Click on the box for 'Display drawing guides on screen' and hit 'OK'.

!!!!!!!!!!!!!!!!!! *Note !*   With older versions of PowerPoint, type 'Ctrl G' to display or hide guides.

The default guides include one vertical and one horizontal and they intersect at the screen center.

With the guides visible, select the logo and move it to the left and then back again towards the center. The logo should snap to the vertical guide, making it easy to ensure alignment (Fig. 7.4).

Figure 7.3
Align Center command.

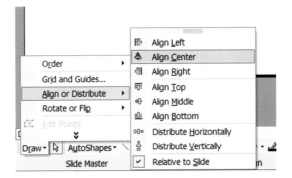

Figure 7.4
Vertical alignment using guides.

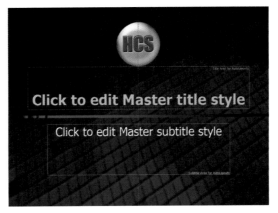

With the logo selected, type 'Ctrl C' to copy it to the clipboard. Hit the 'Page Up' key (or navigate using the arrows in the lower right) to go to the Slide Master. Type 'Ctrl V' to paste the logo and then double-click on it to bring up the 'Format Picture' dialogue box. The logo needs to be a bit smaller for this layout, so click the 'Size' tab and change one dimension to '45%'. And lastly, move the logo to the upper right corner of the slide (Fig. 7.5).

Figure 7.5
Slide Master with logo in position.

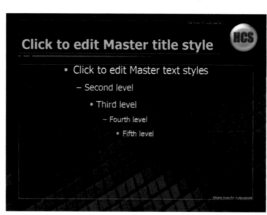

Select 'Close Master View' from the Slide Master dialogue box to switch to slide view.

!!!!!!!!!!!!!!!! Note !   In older versions of PowerPoint, select View > Normal.

Select File > Save As, select 'Presentation' as the type of file, and type 'HCS' (or whatever you wish) and choose 'Save'.

Insert a picture

Chapter 4 described how to resize your image in Photoshop Elements and why you should do so before inserting it into your presentation. Photoshop gives you much better control over your images, and how they will appear in PowerPoint.

Type Ctrl M (or select Insert > New Slide). The new slide will default to the Slide Master set-up, with the Title and Text placeholders. Select and delete the Text placeholder for now.

!!!!!!!!!!!!!!!! Note !   You can always select Format > Slide Layout and choose the Title only layout, but this requires more steps and more time.

Select Insert > Picture > From File, navigate to the Chapter 7 folder on the CD and double-click 'Peutz-Jegher.jpg.'

!!!!!!!!!!!!!!!! Note !   This image is reproduced with permission, you must not remove the copyright link to the website.

The image will be inserted in the center of the slide. Hit the down-arrow key on your keyboard to move the image underneath the blue line. Notice that the image size works perfectly on the slide layout. This is because it was sized to 500 pixels wide.

Type in the Title area 'Peutz-Jegher Syndrome' and type 'Ctrl S' to save your presentation (Fig. 7.6).

Figure 7.6
Insert picture from file.

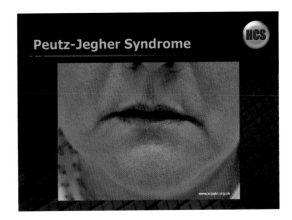

Picture toolbar

The 'Picture' toolbar in PowerPoint includes some tools that you may wish to use with your images. If the Picture toolbar does not automatically appear when you select a picture, right-click on an image and select 'Show Picture Toolbar' (Fig. 7.7).

Figure 7.7
Picture toolbar
in PowerPoint 2002.

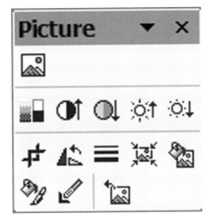

We will only describe a few of these tools. Complete instructions for using each tool can be found in the 'Help' section included with your PowerPoint software. The middle row of tools includes functions for adjusting color, contrast and brightness.

In the next row down you will find the 'Crop' tool. This tool can be very useful when developing your presentation, especially when you only want to trim a small section of your image.

In PowerPoint 2002, you can rotate any picture. Click and drag the green circle (rotation handle) at the top of your picture to rotate freely. Click the 'Rotate left' icon in the Picture Toolbar to rotate your picture 90° counter-clockwise.

Also new to PowerPoint 2002 is image compression. You can compress any image, thus reducing your PowerPoint file size. When selecting the 'Compress Pictures' icon from the Picture Toolbar, you can choose between 'Print resolution at 200 dpi' (if your original image happens to be a higher

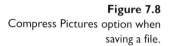

Figure 7.8
Compress Pictures option when saving a file.

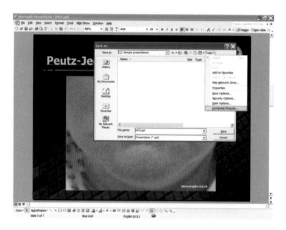

resolution) and 'Web/screen resolution at 96 dpi'. Another option with this tool is to 'Delete cropped areas of pictures'. This will also decrease your file size.

PowerPoint 2002 also allows you to compress all of the images in your presentation in one step. You can find this feature under File > Save As; select the 'Tools' tab and then 'Compress Pictures' (Fig. 7.8). Because you have little control over this tool in PowerPoint, we strongly recommend saving an original copy of your presentation as back-up, prior to compressing pictures.

The 'Reset Picture' icon (in the lower right corner of the Picture toolbar) comes in very handy if you have incorrectly scaled, squashed, or distorted your image in PowerPoint. Click this icon to restore the image to its original settings.

Borders and shadows

You might want to add a border or a drop shadow to your images. This is not always desired or necessary, but can be a design element in your presentation.

On the 'Peutz-Jegher Syndrome' slide that you just completed, select the picture, and click the black arrow next to 'Line Color' in the center of the bottom toolbar. Choose a medium blue (there is a blue swatch in the top of the color palette). The border will default to a setting of 2¼ pt. You can change this by selecting another style from the 'Line Style' icon (on the bottom toolbar, near the center) (Figs 7.9 and 7.10).

You can also elect to add a drop shadow by selecting the 'Shadow Style' icon from the bottom toolbar as well. Select 'Shadow Settings' to bring up the toolbar for editing (Figs 7.11 and 7.12).

The settings on this toolbar allow you to format shadow color and to move it slightly in each direction (nudge). Just for practice, add a drop shadow, change some of the settings and type 'Ctrl S' to save your results.

Aligning multiple pictures

On many occasions, you will need to insert more than one image on a slide. You want the images to be lined up and you want them spaced evenly. How do you align and distribute the images properly?

Figure 7.9
Line Colors tool.

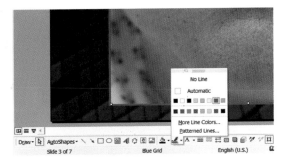

Figure 7.10
Line Styles tool.

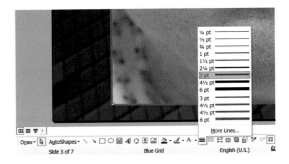

Figure 7.11
Shadow Style icon.

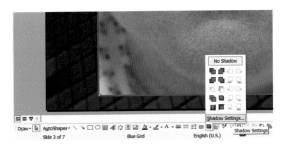

Figure 7.12
Shadow Settings toolbar.

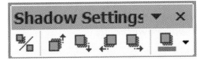

Type 'Ctrl M' (or Insert > New Slide). Delete the text placeholder and type in the title 'X-ray images'. Select Insert > Picture > From File, navigate to the Chapter 7 folder and double-click on the file 'dislocation.jpg'. Drag the image over to the left side of the slide. Select Insert > Picture > From File and double-click on the file 'elbow.jpg'. Lastly, insert the picture 'chest.jpg' and move it anywhere on the right side of the slide.

With the 'Snap to Grid' function turned on, it is fairly simple to align the top of these three images. We will teach you how to align and distribute them using PowerPoint tools.

Hold down the 'Shift' key, and click on each image to select them all (or you can click and drag a selection box around them, whichever is easier

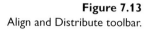

Figure 7.13
Align and Distribute toolbar.

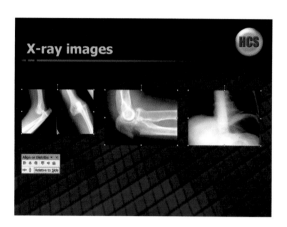

for you). Click the Draw button in the lower left corner and navigate to Align or Distribute.

!!!!!!!!!!!!!!!!!! *Tip* !   Hold your cursor over the top of this fly-out menu; when it turns blue you can 'peel' it off and drag it anywhere onto your screen for quick access.

Click the icon for 'Align Top', then 'Relative to Slide', and finally 'Distribute Horizontally' (Fig. 7.13).

!!!!!!!!!!!!!!!!!! *Tip* !   Briefly hold your cursor on any icon to see its name.

Use the 'Align and Distribute' tools to align text, shapes and images throughout your presentation.

Pick up and apply

Now, we want to use the same outline and drop shadow settings as the previous slide. You could write down these settings and follow the steps each time you add a new image. However, there is a much faster and easier way to accomplish this using the 'Pick up and Apply Object Style' eye-droppers.

!!!!!!!!!!!!!!!!!! *Note* !   This could be one of the most useful efficiency tips you will ever learn for working with PowerPoint!

Select Tools > Customize, and select the 'Commands' tab. Choose the 'Format' category on the left side and scroll down the 'Commands' menu on the right side until you see 'Pick Up Object Style'. Click and drag the eye-dropper icon until it locks into place on your bottom toolbar. Do the same with the 'Apply to Defaults' icon. You will only need to do this once; the icons will appear in position the next time you open PowerPoint (Fig. 7.14).

!!!!!!!!!!!!!!!!!! *Note* !   The dark vertical bar (looks like a capital 'I') will appear where you are going to place the icon. It must be inserted on an existing toolbar, not over the gray background (Fig. 7.15).

Now that your eye-droppers are within easy reach, hit the 'Page Up' key to return to the first image slide. Select the picture (formatted with an outline and drop shadow) and click the 'Pick Up Object Style' icon (Fig. 7.16).

Figure 7.14
Customize Commands
dialogue box.

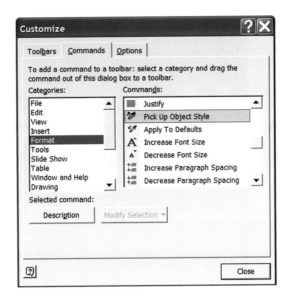

Figure 7.15
Insert a new command icon
onto a toolbar.

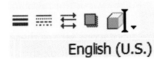

Figure 7.16
Pick Up Object Style command.

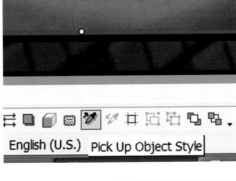

Figure 7.17
Apply Object Style command.

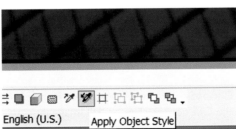

Hit the 'Page Down' key to advance to the X-ray images slide, select all three pictures (by holding the shift key), and then click the 'Apply Object Style' icon. Type 'Ctrl S' to save (Fig. 7.17).

These 'eye-dropper' tools will pick up and apply fill styles, line styles, and text formatting. The last object style you 'picked-up' will remain in memory

Figure 7.18
Aligned images with outlines and
drop shadows.

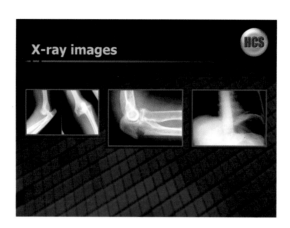

ready to apply to another object until you pick up another style. So you can continue creating slides, and still apply these same attributes later on in your presentation. You can also jump from slide to slide whenever necessary, picking up attributes from one slide and applying them to an object on another slide. And – they work the same in older versions of PowerPoint (Fig. 7.18).

There are many more icons where these came from. If you want to speed up your work even more, look through the 'Customize Commands' dialogue box and customize your toolbars with icons for your favorite tools.

Fill shape with a picture

Filling a shape with a picture is not something you will need for every presentation. Consider it a design option, learn how to accomplish this effectively and file it away for future reference.

Type 'Ctrl M' (Insert > New Slide) and delete the text placeholder. Click on the 'Oval' autoshape icon from the bottom toolbar, place your cursor near the center of the slide, hold down the 'Ctrl' and 'Shift' keys, click and drag a large circle.

! ! ! ! ! ! ! ! ! ! ! ! ! ! ! ! ! ! ! Note !

Holding down the 'Ctrl' key starts the oval from the center, holding the 'Shift' key constrains the circle to even proportions.

With the circle selected, click on the 'Apply Object Style' icon (eye-dropper) to add the outline and drop shadow. Next, click the black arrow next to the 'Fill Color' icon on the bottom toolbar and select 'Fill Effects'. Choose the 'Picture' tab, 'Select Picture', navigate to the Chapter folder on the CD, double-click on 'Fill Image.jpg', and hit 'OK'. Type 'Ctrl S' to save.

This effect will only work properly if your shape and image are in the same proportions. If your image is rectangular, you can easily crop it into an even square using Photoshop Elements. Resave this square image with a new file name and use it to fill a proportionately even shape. If you choose to fill a rectangle or oval, or some other shape with uneven sides, keep the proportions the same (1×3, 2×4, 3×5, etc.). If you don't, your image will appear stretched or squashed (Fig. 7.19).

Figure 7.19
Circle filled with picture
(photography by Royal College
of Surgeons Photographic
Studios).

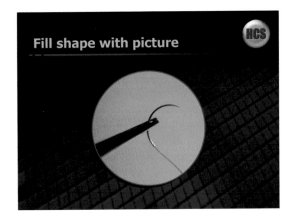

Figure 7.20
Picture fill background.

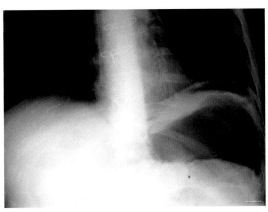

Fill background with picture

In certain cases, an image will speak for itself and you want to fill the background entirely. To ensure the best quality, make sure your image is the same size as your display settings (800 × 600, 1024 × 768 pixels, or other).

! ! ! ! ! ! ! ! ! ! ! ! ! ! ! ! ! Note !

Remember that the display settings refer to the system that will be used during the actual presentation. If quality is an important issue, it is always better to ask first and set your display settings accordingly.

Once again use 'Ctrl M' to open a new slide and delete both placeholders. Right-click anywhere on the slide, and select 'Background' (Format > Background) and check the box next to 'Omit background graphics from Master'. Next, click the small black arrow near the center, 'Fill Effects', then the 'Picture' tab. Select 'Picture' and from the chapter folder double-click the file 'X-ray.jpg'. Click 'OK' and finally 'Apply'. The X-ray image is 1024 × 768 pixels. Type 'Ctrl S' to save your sample presentation (Fig. 7.20).

Insert movies

Movies are digital video files with formats like '.mov', '.avi', and '.mpg', to name a few. As technology advances at its rapid pace, these digital videos are becoming more and more common. It is relatively easy to insert a movie into your presentation but some file formats require playing through the Windows® Media Player to work properly. It is always best to test your movie early and, if you run into any problems, refer to the Help feature in PowerPoint or the Microsoft PowerPoint website for more information.

This time choose Insert > Movies and sounds > Movie from file. Navigate to PET.mpg in the Chapter 7 folder (this movie file was kindly donated by Dr Gary Cook at the Guys and St. Thomas' PET Centre, London, UK). Insert this. You will be asked if you want the movie to play automatically – in this case we do, so click 'Yes'. If you want the movie to start on a mouse click, choose 'No'.

We want the movie to repeat continuously until the next mouse click. Right-click on the movie image and select Edit > Movie Object, and then check the box next to 'Loop until stopped'. Type 'Ctrl S' to save the presentation. Preview this slide by selecting the Slide Show icon from the lower left corner of your screen (Fig. 7.21).

Figure 7.21
PET.mpg (courtesy of the PET Centre, Guys & St Thomas Hospital, London).

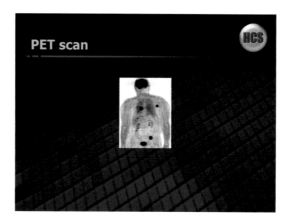

Notice that the movie is relatively small in relation to the slide area. That is because the movie dimensions are small (roughly 200 pixels in height). We do not recommend stretching the image in PowerPoint to make the movie larger, as ultimately this will affect the quality of your movie and can cause playback to slow down.

The file size of a movie is directly affected by its dimensional size. A larger-sized movie will consist of more megabytes and might slow down during playback. If you are going to be using a lot of digital video, make sure you have sufficient memory and a good quality video card.

Movies and sounds are linked to your PowerPoint file. The best way to work with movie and sound files is to copy them into your working folder, the same folder as your PowerPoint file, and then insert them onto your slides. You *must* copy the movie and sound files along with your PowerPoint file for playing on another system. PowerPoint does not embed large sound files, or any movie file (another reason for you to consider your movie file size). If you insert the movie from the same folder as your presentation, it will play properly when both files are copied to another system. Inserting and playing movies is a difficult issue in PowerPoint. Have a look at the website for additional help.

There are more options available for playing movies and adding sound in PowerPoint. If this interests you, refer to the PowerPoint Help section 'Creating Presentations – Adding Sound, Music, Video, and Voice'.

PowerPoint 2002 Photo Album

PowerPoint 2002 includes a terrific new feature, called 'Photo Album', which will automatically place images into a new presentation. The Photo Album tool works great for creating presentations from an entire folder of digital images. You can use it to develop a quick, image-intensive show or use it to compile your latest digital camera images into one file for review.

Select File > Close to close out the previous presentation. Select Insert > Picture > New Photo Album. This will bring up the Photo Album dialogue box (Fig. 7.22).

Next, choose 'Insert picture from File/Disk' and navigate to the 'Photo Album' folder inside the chapter folder. Click to highlight the top file in the list: 'Image01', hold down the 'Shift' key and click on the bottom file in the list: 'Image04' and select 'Insert'.

!!!!!!!!!!!!!!!!! Note !

Holding down the Shift key will highlight everything in between the first and last selection.

Within the Photo Album dialogue box are options for rotation, brightness and contrast, and adding a text box. You also have various 'Album Layouts' to choose from: 'Fit to slide', '2 pictures', '4 pictures', and so on. Keep this setting on 'Fit to slide' and select 'Create'.

Almost instantly, you have an opening slide (edit or delete it, your choice) and four, full-frame image slides. You can add captions, program transitions, and you are all finished with your digital 'Photo Album' (Fig. 7.23).

Figure 7.22
Photo Album dialogue box.

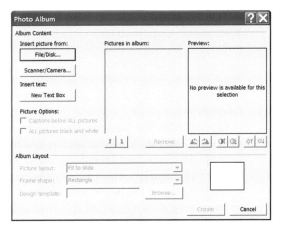

Figure 7.23
Slide Sorter view of Photo Album.

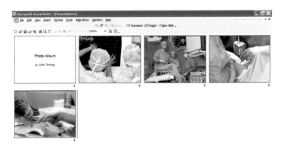

Figure 7.24
Highlighted cells from
Excel® spreadsheet.

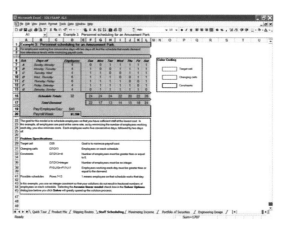

Figure 7.25
Excel table, Paste Options in
PowerPoint.

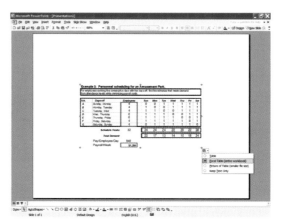

Copying an Excel spreadsheet to PowerPoint

You might be giving a talk that relates to some research or management work involving a spreadsheet in Excel. How can you copy from this program to PowerPoint?

Open the file 'SolvSamp.xls' from the chapter folder. In fact, if you have Excel on your PC you will have this file; it is one of the sample files supplied with the program. Click the 'Staff Scheduling' tab at the bottom of your screen.

You need to select only the information you wish to copy into PowerPoint. Keep the left mouse button pressed and drag a box encompassing cells A1 to L20; this will highlight the table at the top of the spreadsheet. Type 'Ctrl C' to copy this selection to the clipboard (Fig. 7.24).

Switch to PowerPoint and type 'Ctrl V' to paste the data onto a blank slide. Notice that the table is stretched vertically and does not look like the original from Excel. You will see a small clipboard in the lower right corner of the table; click on the icon to see your 'Paste Options'.

The radio button for 'Table' is automatically selected. This causes the Excel table to be stretched vertically on your slide.

If you choose 'Excel Table (entire workbook)' your table will be reformatted as it appears in Excel (Fig. 7.25). Plus, it will be fully editable, which is very important if your data will be changing. This is the best choice of all the Paste Options. Click and drag to highlight any set of cells, then

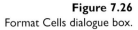
Figure 7.26
Format Cells dialogue box.

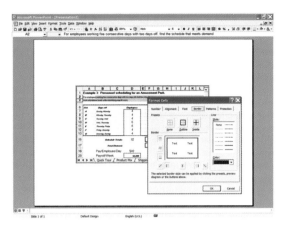

right-click and choose 'Format Cells' to change fonts, sizes, borders, fills, alignment, etc. (Fig. 7.26).

The next selection, 'Picture of Table (smaller file size)', will paste the table onto the slide as a picture. In this instance, the table is not that complicated to begin with, so the file size has not decreased dramatically. This option might be useful in a few instances where your table is very complex, but for most purposes you should choose 'Excel Table'.

The last choice, 'Keep Text Only', converts the entire table to text. This is not desirable for our example, but you never know when you may need this particular option.

Chapter 8

Preparing images for use on the internet

Jason Smith and Terry Irwin

If you are not interested in website design you might think this chapter is irrelevant to you. You are wrong! Why would a healthcare professional want or need to put images on the web? There are several reasons:

■ Producing a website is also relatively easy. Many internet service providers (ISPs) provide online tools to develop a basic site. If you have a POP3 e-mail account (i.e. not an account like Hotmail or MSN) you probably have free web space for you to make your own site.
■ You might want to develop a patient or professional education/information site. Although someone else might design it, you will need to send them images.
■ You might decide to store images on the web, either for safekeeping or so that colleagues, friends, or family can access them.
■ You might access a newsgroup and want to add images to your messages.
■ You might decide to put your presentation on the web.

The final point might seem a little strange but with increasing numbers of institutions having computers connected to the web, online presentation is a real and exciting possibility allowing more flexibility than PowerPoint® currently offers. If your images are too large (in terms of file size) the presentation will be very slow to download and show, especially over a slow connection, and readers will lose interest.

There are undoubtedly many reasons, other than those listed above, and this chapter aims to provide some fundamental concepts of how images are presented and manipulated for web usage and how best to optimize them.

Although we want you to understand how images are used on the web, you really don't need to know all of this; however, it might stimulate you to learn more.

Serving an image to the web browser

When web servers were first prototyped, they 'served' simple HTML documents and images. Image use on the web has been popular since the very first browser (NCSA Mosaic) was released in 1993.

So what does a web server do? In its most basic form it sends static content to a web browser on the user's computer. This means that the web server receives a request for a web page such as: http://www.aesgbi.org/index.php (Fig. 8.1). The server then maps that uniform resource locator (URL) to a local file on the host server, that is, it looks to see which file the URL refers to and where it is stored on the server.

Figure 8.1
A typical web page.

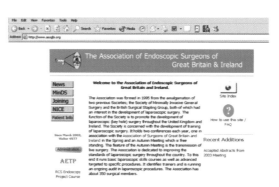

In this case, the file 'index.php' is somewhere on the host file system. The server then loads this file and sends it to the user's web browser. This entire exchange is mediated by the browser and server talking to each other using hypertext transfer protocol (HTTP) language (Fig. 8.2).

Figure 8.2
The relationship between a web browser, web server, and the file that is being displayed.

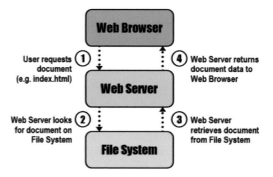

This simple arrangement, which allows the serving of static content such as hypertext markup language (HTML) and image files to a web browser, was the initial concept behind what we now call the worldwide web.

Fundamentally, an image embedded in a web page is interpreted as a string of binary data (1s and 0s). The higher the 'quality' of the image the more data there is to embed, and the longer it will take to download from the web server to your web browser and be displayed on your screen. Resolution of images was covered in detail in an earlier chapter but will be briefly covered in this chapter with specific reference to the web.

Dedicated image servers are available as a single-source image repository. With this type of server each image is saved in just one format. Special URLs are then inserted as hyperlinks into the HTML to serve up all of the variations from a single image: render in different formats, change size, pan, zoom, and change color, and so on. Effectively, all processing is done 'on-the-fly' by the server and the required result sent to the user's browser. This avoids the need to have several copies of the same image in different formats, sizes, and so on, depending on the intended use.

Image formats for use on the web

Most web browsers above the fourth generation (Internet Explorer 4 (IE4), Netscape 4, etc.) will display a variety of image formats such as .bmp, .jpeg, .gif, and .png. There is little point using a bitmap (.bmp) image on the web because the file size is too large and download times will be excessive. The most common image formats on the web are GIF and JPEG.

GIF images

You already know that GIFs support up to 8 bits per pixel, which means a maximum of 256 colors. This format is the most commonly used image format on the web and includes features that enable background transparency and animation. GIF is an image format that uses a compression algorithm (Lempel-Ziv Welch compression algorithm, or LZW) to reduce the file size of the image and hence speed-up download times. The LZW compression algorithm is a form of lossless compression. This is based on the idea of breaking a file into a 'smaller' form for transmission or storage and then putting it back together at the other end so it can be used again. It is called lossless compression because it lets you recreate the original file exactly. Remember that the LZW algorithm was not designed for photographic images and does not work well with true-color images. It is best used for images with few colors, such as cartoon graphics and transparent images.

JPEG images

JPEG is not actually a file format; rather it is a compression algorithm that produces a JFIF image (JPEG File Interchange Format). The type of compression is different from that used in GIF images in that it uses lossy compression. The algorithm simply eliminates 'unnecessary' bits of information. JPEG is designed to exploit certain properties of our eyes; namely, that we are more sensitive to slow changes of brightness and color than we are to rapid changes over a short distance. This type of compression is often used for reducing the file size of bitmap pictures, which tend to be fairly large. JPEGs work well on continuous tone images like photographs but not so well on sharp-edged or flat-color art like lettering, simple cartoons, or line drawings. JPEGs support 24-bits of color depth or 16.7 million colors.

To understand lossy compression, consider a scanned image of a scene, half of which is filled with a blue sky. Lossless compression algorithms can do very little with this type of image. Whereas large parts of the picture look the same – the whole sky is blue, for example – most of the individual pixels are a little bit different. To make this picture smaller without compromising the resolution, you have to change the color value for certain pixels. If the picture had a lot of blue sky, the algorithm would pick one color of blue that could be used for every pixel. Then, the algorithm rewrites the file so that

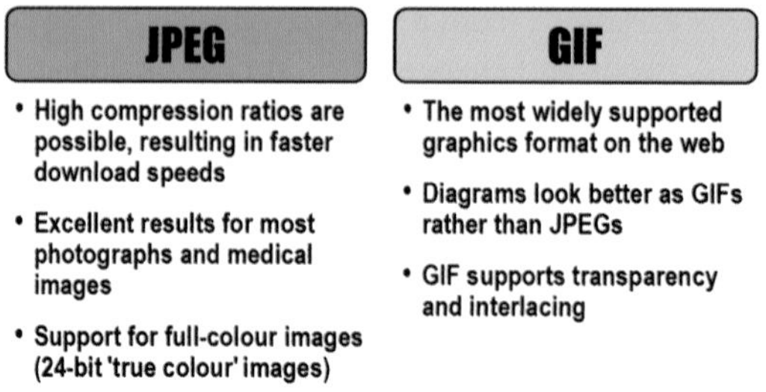

Figure 8.3
Choosing a GIF or a JPEG.

JPEG	GIF
• High compression ratios are possible, resulting in faster download speeds	• The most widely supported graphics format on the web
• Excellent results for most photographs and medical images	• Diagrams look better as GIFs rather than JPEGs
• Support for full-colour images (24-bit 'true colour' images)	• GIF supports transparency and interlacing

the value for every sky pixel refers back to this information. If the compression scheme works well, you won't notice the change but the file size will be significantly reduced. The greater the degree of compression the more noticeable the change is compared to the original. Overcompressing a JPEG file leads to a grainy, blurred and distorted image.

! ! ! ! ! ! ! ! ! ! ! ! ! ! ! ! ! ! ! Note !   You cannot reverse or 'put back' the compression, hence the reason for doing image manipulation before applying compression.

PNG images

PNG was designed as a replacement for GIF as there were certain legal wrangles with respect to copyright and royalties from CompuServe and Unisys, who originated the format. A good summary for those who are interested can be found at http://www.pwr.wroc.pl/AMIGA/AR/ar304_Sections/feature2.html

PNG is an extensible file format for the lossless, portable, well-compressed storage of raster images (such as bitmaps). PNG provides a patent-free replacement for GIF and can also replace many common uses of TIFF. Indexed-color, grayscale (16 bits), and true-color (48 bits) images are supported, plus an optional alpha channel, thereby improving on the transparency features of GIFs. The PNG format does not support multiple images (animation). Although PNG is a better format it has been slow to catch on with web designers due to the dominance of the GIF format.

JPEG or GIF – that is the question!

The simple answer to this is: 'Lots of colors = JPEG … Solid colors or no gradations = GIF'.

Remember, both GIF and JPEG image formats are compression based. The usual result of this conversion is a significantly smaller image size. It might seem that one compression method would always result in smaller file sizes, but that is simply not the case (Fig. 8.3).

If in doubt, save your images in both formats, examine the file sizes and what the images look like when opened in a browser such as Internet Explorer, then make a decision as to which is best for your purposes.

Image manipulation for use on the web

Let us assume you have scanned a color photograph at 72 dpi for publication on a web page. Some optimization is required to get the best results. All image editing should be done on the raw scanned file before saving as a compressed file as the results will be much better.

Figure 8.4
Most monitors are
800 × 600, so web pages are
resolved to this setting.

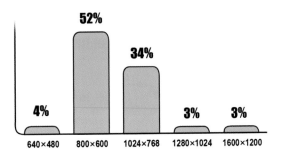

monitor resolution for web browsing

The first thing to do is crop the image to include only what you require. If you are unsure how to do this, refer to Chapter 14.

The image can now be adjusted to enhance the appearance. Images for the web are usually small and low resolution, so simple fixes are all that is needed in most cases. This is best done with the 'Quick Fix' option in Photoshop Elements®. Choose 'Enhance' from the main menu and then 'Quick Fix'. This gives you multiple options to improve the levels, hue, saturation, brightness, and so on, with a preview image before the changes are applied.

Now resize your image to the dimensions you require by choosing Image > Resize > Image Size. By default, height and width are constrained so altering one alters the other proportionately. This can be turned off if necessary by unchecking the relevant box. Images for the web are tiny compared to images used in print media or in PowerPoint. For example, many images on the web will be as small as 120 × 80 pixels, which at 72 dpi will make the file about 25 kilobytes in size. Compare this with the original image, which might be 20 times the physical dimensions and resolution and as much as 500 times the file size.

Remember that the image must be optimized for the most common size of monitor (Fig. 8.4), not the one the designer is using. Most people still feel that web pages should be optimized for 800 × 600 pixels, so a 200-pixel-wide image will occupy one-quarter of the screen.

One of the advantages of Photoshop Elements is the 'Save for the web' feature (File > Save For Web). There are several options to choose from here, including the type of image and color palette used. Experiment with these and look at the preview image supplied to determine what is best for your use. The added advantage of this system is that the preview image also specifies the file size and estimated download time on a modem that receives 28.8 kilobytes per second, the slowest commonly available modem. Of course, if you are *certain* that all your users will have 56-kilobyte per second modems or T1 lines, you can allow for higher speed downloads.

Transparent background images

It might be necessary to create your images with transparent backgrounds. An example of this might be when you want a logo to 'float' on a different color background. The easy way is to include a transparent layer when you first create the image and make sure that the box for transparency is

Figure 8.5
Transparency in a web logo.

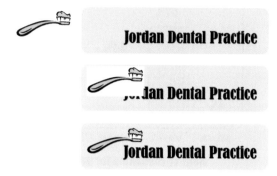

checked in the 'Save for web' dialog box. There are two options for this. If you select transparency, partially transparent pixels are filled with the matte color specified in the drop-down list, and fully transparent pixels remain transparent. When you place the image on a web page, the edges of the image blend with the background, which shows through the fully transparent pixels. This option prevents the halo effect that results when you place an anti-aliased image on a web page background that differs from the image background. This option also prevents the jagged edges of hard-edged transparency. If you deselect transparency, fully transparent pixels are filled with the matte color and partially transparent pixels are blended with the matte color. The harder way (beyond the scope of this chapter) is to create a transparent alpha channel to allow the background of the page to 'come through'. However, if you use a .png file this is not an issue (Fig. 8.5).

Basic HTML for including images on web pages

We are not going try to teach you HTML – there are many books and internet resources available on this subject. This section simply introduces the <img> tag and how you can use it to modify how your images are displayed.

That said, let's learn a little HTML – OK we lied, but just a little! Don't be put off, it will be easy and you might even enjoy it. All of the HTML examples below can be viewed on the web by going to http://www. perfectmedicalpresentations.com and choosing the appropriate example. When a page loads, if you want to confirm that we have used this code, select View > Source in your browser.

Example 1

Open Notepad (Start > All Programs > Accessories > Notepad). Type the following text in to the document.

```
<html>
<head>
<title> My first go at html </title>
</head>
<body>
</body>
</html>
```

This tells the browser to look at this file as an 'HTML' (hypertext markup language) document. The header gives some very basic information – this document is called 'My first go at HTML'. This is the text that will show along the top of your browser when the page loads. There is nothing in the document yet, but the content will go in the body, just as the text of a report goes in the correct place.

Example 2

Now we will add some text. Type something after the word 'body'. The < /head > and < /body > tell the browser that this line is the end of the head or body sections. Your document might look like this:

```
<html>
<head>
<title> My first go at html </title>
</head>
<body>
This is my first attempt to write html. I have no real
idea what I am doing, but I am learning.
I do not know how to make a paragraph yet, but I am
willing to learn that too!
</body>
</html>
```

Now save the file to your desktop. Select File > Save As, change 'Save As' type to 'All Files', and then type in the file name 'first.html'. Now look on the desktop. Amazing! The file you created now looks like it is a web page – it has the same icon as any other web page. That is because Windows® recognizes your instruction that this is HTML!

Now open it by double-clicking it. The file opens in your default web browser and should look like the examples on the Perfect Medical Presentations website.

Example 3

Note that you really do not know how to do paragraphs yet! So, go back to Notepad and change the text to this:

```
<html>
<head>
<title> My first go at html </title>
</head>
<body>
<p> This is my first attempt to write html. I have no
real idea what I am doing, but I am learning. </p>
<p> Now I can even make a paragraph </p>
</body>
</html>
```

Save this file to your desktop as 'second.html'. Now open it from the desktop and note that the instruction <p> means 'I am starting a paragraph' and `</p>` means 'I am ending a paragraph'. OK, that is enough basic HTML, what about images?

In its simplest form the `<img>` tag tells the browser to place an image at the current location in the HTML document being displayed in the browser. The tag uses the following format to display the image: `<img src='emma.jpg'>`. This tells the browser that it is to show an image and that the image source (src) is a file called 'emma', which is a jpeg file located in the same place, that is, in the same directory as the page it is reading.

You need to remember that some people will browse with 'images turned off' for a number of reasons. This is less of a problem these days but your web page should conform to accepted usability standards and needs to be designed so that the maximum number of people can view it adequately. Good usability states that all images should have the 'alt' tag modifier included as such:

```
<img src='emma.jpg' alt='Emma's eye'>
```

Adding alt tags might seem a bit advanced for us here but to see it in action, just hold your mouse over an image on a web page – the alt tag is the text that appears. Adding the 'alt' modifier to the `<img>` tag allows the browser to display the text message (enclosed in quotes) when the mouse pointer hovers over the image or instead of the image if the user has turned images off.

Look at the first part of the above piece of HTML in detail, `<img src='emma.jpg'>` specifies the file name of the image to be displayed and also its relative location to the current document. As just a file name is displayed, HTML assumes that the image is located in the same folder as the current document on the web server. If you want to specify an alternative location you need to be specific such as:

```
<img src='images/emma.jpg'> or <img src='./images/emma.jpg'>
```

These might seem confusing at first because they specify the 'path' to the file as recognized by the web servers. The former tells the browser to look for the filename 'emma.jpg' in the directory 'images' that lies within the current directory. The latter tells the browser to come out of the current directory (as in go up a level) and then look for a directory called 'images' in which the file 'emma.jpg' is located. You can also use absolute paths specifying the full URL to the file as well. More detail on directory structure can be found in most standard texts on HTML programing.

Example 4

So let's add an image to your web page. Save the image 'emma.jpg' (which is in the Chapter 8 folder on the CD) onto your computer desktop giving it the name 'image.jpg'. Note that it is about 200 pixels wide. Now modify the text in Notepad to say this:

```
<html>
<head>
<title> My first go at html </title>
</head>
```

```
<body>
<p> This is my first attempt to write html. I have no
real idea what I am doing, but I am learning. </p>
<p> Now I can even make a paragraph </p>
<img src='image.jpg' alt='Golly it works!'>
</body>
</html>
```

Save it as 'third.html' on your desktop. Always save as the file type .html and always change the file type to 'All Files'. If the alt does not work, it is because you are using smart quotations, as in Word. You must use the very basic quotations in NotePad.

Now open this document using your browser. Look, an image! Now hold your mouse over the image to see the alt tag modifier.

Example 5   Now for the really clever bit. Your image does not even need to be your own image! Change the text in Notepad to say this:

```
<html>
<head>
<title> My first go at html </title>
</head>
<body>
<p> This is my first attempt to write html. I have no
real idea what I am doing, but I am learning. </p>
<p> Now I can even make a paragraph </p>
<img src='http://www.perfectmedicalpresentations.com/
images/bodyimage1.jpg' alt='This is on the book web site!'>
</body>
</html>
```

The instruction: `<img src='http://www.perfectmedical presentations.com/images/bodyimage1.jpg' alt='This is on the book web site!'>` tells the browser to look for the image on another server, in this case the website for this book. 'Netiquette' (acceptable practice on the internet) does discourage this though (see Chapter 9 for an explanation). Naturally, we are very happy for you to link to the website. Of course, your computer needs to be connected to the internet for this command to work.

Save the file as before and then open it. Now you are an expert at HTML! There are many other `<img>` tag modifiers and these are described briefly in the table in Figure 8.6.

Most people will not need to consider raw coding of HTML because they will use a WYSIWYG (what you see is what you get) editor such as Macromedia Dreamweaver or Microsoft FrontPage to build the web pages. Nevertheless, it is useful to know what the tags do and how to manipulate them, as WYSIWYG editors don't always give WYSIWYG results!

There are other reasons to learn a little HTML in relation to images. For example, many bulletin boards will let you add images to your posted

Figure 8.6
Alternative tag modifiers.

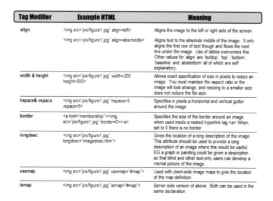

Tag Modifier	Example HTML	Meaning
align	\<img src="pix/figure1.jpg" align=left>	Aligns the image to the left or right side of the screen
	\<img src="pix/figure1.jpg" align=absmiddle>	Aligns text to the absolute middle of the image. It only aligns the first row of text though and flows the next line under the image. Use of tables overcomes this. Other values for 'align' are 'texttop', 'top', 'bottom', 'baseline' and 'absbottom' all of which are self explanatory.
width & height	\<img src="pix/figure1.jpg" width=200 height=300>	Allows exact specification of size in pixels to resize an image. You must maintain the aspect ratio or the image will look strange, and resizing to a smaller size does not reduce the file size.
hspace& vspace	\<img src="pix/figure1.jpg" hspace=5 vspace=5>	Specifies in pixels a horizontal and vertical gutter around the image
border	\<a href="membership/">\<img src="pix/figure1.jpg" border=0></a>	Specifies the size of the border around an image when used inside a nested hyperlink tag \<a> When set to 0 there is no border.
longdesc	\<img src="pix/figure1.jpg" longdesc="imagedesc.htm">	Gives the location of a long description of the image. This attribute should be used to provide a long description of an image where this would be useful. EG a graph or painting could be given a description so that blind and other text-only users can develop a mental picture of the image.
usemap	\<img src="pix/figure1.jpg" usemap="#map">	Used with client-side image maps to give the location of the map definition.
ismap	\<img src="pix/figure1.jpg" ismap="#map">	Server side version of above. Both can be used in the same declaration

messages. To do this you need to use appropriate code for the board. The most common is Ultimate Bulletin Board™ (UBB), indeed that is what is used on www. perfectmedicalpresentations.com. To learn the UBB commands click on the word BB code to the left of the message box when you are posting (Fig. 8.7) and follow the link in the FAQs to 'Can you please explain the BB code to me?'.

Figure 8.7
Where to find information on using UBB code.

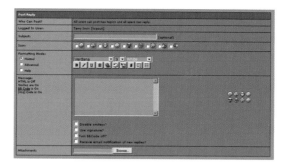

If you want to know the URL of an image on a web page, go to the website that contains it and right-click over the image that you want to use. Choose 'properties' and highlight the text after the heading 'address URL.' This goes in place of http://www.mysite.com/images/picture.gif in the above instruction. You can add your own alt command using `alt='This is where the alt text goes!'>`, as in the example above.

Why not try posting a message on the bulletin board at www.perfectmedicalpresentations.com with a link to an image on the site. Choose one that is small so that it will fit on the board.

Image maps

Image maps are areas of your graphic images that are defined as 'hot-spots', allowing hyperlinking to other files or sites. You will have seen these – where an image contains a series of links that you can follow. Image maps are of two varieties: client-side and server-side. Client-side maps are executed by the user's browser, they execute more quickly than server-side image maps because there is no need for the server to process a script. All browsers above the fourth generation support client-side image maps.

We do not want to explore this further here but there are plenty of online tutorials where you can learn how to create image maps.

Uploading the images

You might feel that we have strayed too far from our primary goal already in this chapter! We are definitely not going to get into how you should upload a website. This can be done with some WYSIWYG editors but is best done with a dedicated file transfer protocol (FTP) transfer program such as WS-FTP Pro. You can obtain a copy from the following:
http://www.ipswitch.com/Products/WS_FTP/

The full version has a time-limited trial, but it is well worth buying it. Install and follow the instructions then run the program. You will need the following information from your web host:

- FTP host name
- your username
- your password.

Once you have completed your connection you must remember to upload the files in binary format, not ASCII.

Disclaimers

If you plan to put a large number of images on the web it makes sense to have a disclaimer on the site, clearly visible on every page. Such a suitable disclaimer could look like:

> The graphics, images, and text found on this website, unless stated otherwise, are within the public domain. You can download and use them. Credit back to us is appreciated. If any material is referenced 'Image courtesy of …' or 'Information courtesy of …', then please contact us for permission for use.

Or:

> All words and photographs ©2003 Perfect Medical Presentations unless otherwise stated. All rights reserved. Any use or retransmission of text, images on this website without prior written consent of the copyright owner constitutes copyright infringement and is prohibited.

It is also useful, especially if you are providing a large number of free images, to include the following:

> Please download the images to your own server and do not link directly to the images contained on this site.

The reason for this is that when you link directly to images on other websites it uses bandwidth from the server. If the images are very popular the bandwidth use could crash the server and lead to discontinuation of service. Furthermore, most website hosts charge for a certain volume of bandwidth per month; if you exceed this you will be charged for it.

Preparing a Power Point presentation for the web

You might want to save a PowerPoint presentation for use on the web, perhaps on your own site or on another server. Typically, you might be asked to do this for students after you have given a talk or tutorial. This is very straightforward using PowerPoint.

Open the file 'HCSweb.ppt' from the Chapter 8 folder on the CD. You can preview the web presentation by choosing File > Web Page Preview from

Figure 8.8
Saving a PowerPoint
presentation as HTML.

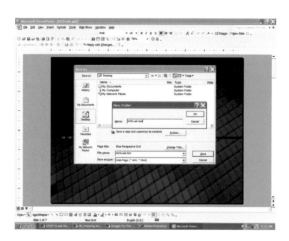

the PowerPoint menu. Now click on 'Slide Show' in the bottom-right corner of the web page that opens. You can click through the slides in order using the left mouse button or the space bar. Close your browser. Remember that websites are not like PowerPoint presentations; you will need to compress your images, and especially any embedded video, otherwise each slide will take a very long time to download and display.

If you like, you can add another one or two slides. When you are happy that the presentation looks fine, choose File > Save as Web Page. Change the 'Save in' selection to your desktop or click on the desktop icon on the left. Click the small icon 'Create new folder' on the top bar and give it the name 'HCSweb test' (Fig. 8.8).

By choosing 'Publish' you can customize the presentation with speaker's notes included or not. The remaining choices are self-explanatory. Now click 'Publish'.

If you now look on your desktop you have a folder called 'HCSweb test', which contains an HTML file called 'HCSweb' and a folder called ' HCSweb_ files'. This folder has all of the files needed for your online presentation.

Open the HTML file 'HCSweb.html'. Note that it looks exactly the same as your original presentation and the preview. However, the animation effects do not work as well in html files – they tend to be a little jerky. The video has been saved in the folder 'HCSweb_files'.

You can now upload these files to your website or send them to the site administrator.

If you have a microphone and a web cam attached to your computer you might like to try preparing a web broadcast. To do so, select Slide Show > Online Broadcast > Record and Save a Broadcast. This is for more advanced users and instructions can be found in the PowerPoint help menus.

Summary

The above covers the basics of image use on the web aimed principally at optimizing presentation with download times. More detail can be found online if you are interested in HTML programming and there is a plethora of books on the subject available online and in street stores.

Chapter 9

Acquiring images from the internet

Jason Smith and Terry Irwin

Before you rush off to download images from the web, remember that most of the images there belong to someone – they will be under copyright. Read the chapter on consent carefully!

There are five potential sources for your images:

- search the web
- screen grabs
- digital photography
- make them yourself in a drawing program
- scanned images.

We will deal with the first two in this chapter.

Searching the web

There are thousands of places to find images on the web – from single pages to dedicated image banks. Once again, the first and most important thing to realize here is that the images might be under copyright and unauthorized use on your web pages or for other purposes could leave you open to prosecution. This will depend on many factors, such as whether the image is in the 'public domain' and if its use is intended for personal, educational, or business purposes. It is useful to consider the following before using images on the web that are not clearly stated as free for all to use:

- don't assume anything
- make every effort to seek written permission from copyright owners before use
- provide appropriate credits for any and all images that you use.

The following web links are good places to start to find images and graphics on the web, although a simple search for free images or free graphics in any of the major search engines will yield plenty of results:

- http://www.webplaces.com/search/
- http://www.google.co.uk/imghp

Note that the standard Google™ search page is not a good way to search for images. Clicking the 'Image' tab will take you to the page shown above.

To save an image from a web page you need to do the following:

- Put your mouse pointer over the image.
- Right click.
- Select 'Save Image As' (Internet Explorer) or 'Save Picture As' (Netscape) from the menu that appears.
- Browse to the folder you want to save the image in.
- Rename the file if necessary.
- Choose 'Save'.

Later versions of Internet Explorer will bring up an icon tray with the options of save, print, email, or open my pictures folder if you just hover over the image. Remember that this image has been optimized for the web. It will be set at 72 dpi and might be only a little over 100 pixels wide. It will look terrible if you try to enlarge it. It might not print very well either. There is very little that you can do about this.

Screen grabs

Screen grabs are fairly easy to do simply by pressing the 'Prnt Scrn' (Print Screen) key on a Windows®-based PC, which copies the screen grab to the clipboard. Using 'Alt-Prnt Scrn' captures only the active window.

We have largely ignored Apple users in this book, because the commands in Photoshop Elements® and in PowerPoint® are so similar (and Mac users generally understand graphics well anyway). However, here there are a few tricks that are not so well known. On a Mac:

- 'Command-Shift-3': captures the entire screen.
- 'Command-Shift-4': pointer turns to cross hair, you specify the area to capture.
- 'Command-Shift-4' (Caps Lock on): bull's eye captures a particular open window.
- 'Command-Shift-4' (Caps Lock on, Control key pressed down before releasing the mouse button): sends screen grab directly to clip board instead of making a Picture (PICT or .PCT) file.

After capturing to the clipboard, you can open the file directly in Photoshop Elements by choosing File > New from Clipboard and your screen grab appears for editing. You can then paste or insert your image into whichever program you are using.

A number of websites contain excellent images for healthcare professionals. Some are free but most require some form of payment. No list can ever be complete, because the web is growing and changing so rapidly. You may want to add your own views on the bulletin boards that complement this book at www.perfectmedicalpresentations.com.

Corbis offer an enormous range of images at www.corbis.com. Most require payment but some are royalty free. For use in PowerPoint, most images will cost less than $10. A similar service is offered by Comstock at

Figure 9.1
www.trauma.org allows
healthcare professionals to use
images for personal use.

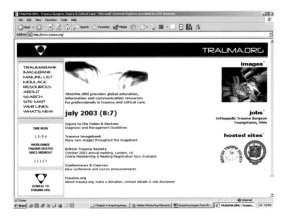

Figure 9.2
A new image bank from
The Royal College of Surgeons
of England.

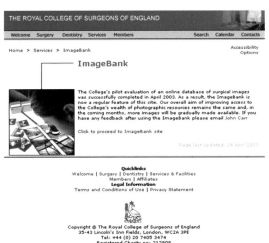

www.comstock.com. A search for 'royalty free medical images' in Google™
will reveal plenty of other sites offering similar services.

Some image sources are completely free as long as use is restricted to
that set out in the terms and conditions. For example, www.trauma.org
allows images to be used for 'personal use' by healthcare professionals only.
It is not suitable for the general public (Fig. 9.1).

The Royal College of Surgeons of England is developing an excellent new
service at http://www.rcseng.ac.uk/services/imagebank/ (Fig. 9.2). Details can
be obtained from jcarr@rcseng.ac.uk.

Of course, you can access free images directly from PowerPoint. Choose
Insert > Picture > Clip Art from the menu. In the bottom-right corner of
the work area you will see a hyperlink to 'Clips Online', which takes you to
the 'Microsoft Office Online' Clip Art and Media website page. Here you can
search for clip art, photos, animations and sound. Choose 'Photos' under the
'Search' menu and type in a key word to search for low resolution, digital
images.

In conclusion, there are lots of excellent resources for you to download
images from the web. Please be sure to stay within the law and do not
'borrow' images without permission.

Chapter 10

Clinical photography

Terry Irwin with contributions from
Joe Niamtu and John Carr

Clinical photographs are an essential part of medical practice, used for teaching and training, as diagnostic aids, as part of the medical record, legal records, marketing tools, and for telemedicine. The clinician who takes lots of images is usually proud of his or her work, enjoys teaching, and is probably therefore a 'good doctor'.

Clinical photography used to be the realm of a select group of interested clinicians and professional photographers, and for many of us, good images were elusive. The professional sometimes failed to capture the essence of the image that we had in mind – perhaps the angle or the crop was not quite right. The reason for this was often our own fault. Proper planning, clear explanation of the purpose of the image, and patience while it was being taken would have helped! However, with careful planning, professional images usually surpass our humble efforts (Fig. 10.1). Trying to 'do it yourself' was complex, requiring considerable practice and expense. Even then, when the images arrived a few days later, they were not always what we had hoped that they would be.

Figure 10.1
Images can capture the essence of the subject. Here the facial expressions tell the story (photography by Royal College of Surgeons Photographic Studios).

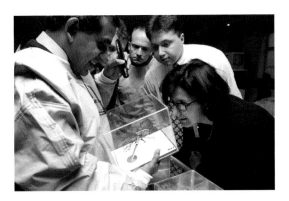

All that has changed with the advent of digital photography; reasonable clinical photography is within the grasp of most interested clinicians. Perhaps the most controversial question is whether a standard digital camera is up to the task, or whether the SLR remains better.

Current 4- to 6-megapixel digital cameras will produce good quality clinical images, suitable for most, although perhaps not all, purposes. For very specialist subjects, a dedicated camera might be needed. The best professional digital cameras are now as good as large-format film cameras. They are very expensive and files are huge, often 20–50 megapixels in size.

For some specialist purposes, for example dental photography, a macro lens and specialist lighting are ideal (Fig. 10.2). Taking an image with a digital camera close to the open mouth usually fails. Furthermore, the flash, if used, will illuminate the skin and not the oral cavity because it is offset from the lens. That is not to say that all intra-oral photography is impossible with a simple digital camera. Using the camera upside down can sometimes illuminate the roof of the mouth sufficiently to give adequate images.

Figure 10.2
Dental images often require specialist lighting and equipment.

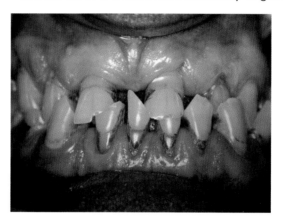

A further problem is parallax error. The view through the viewfinder is fine for distant images but as the photographer moves closer to the subject the two images (that seen through the viewfinder and that read by the CCD) differ. So you aim for the eyes and photograph the mouth and nose! Using the camera display is clearly necessary but accurate focusing can be challenging.

A 6-megapixel camera will provide image files of about 1–5 megabytes each. A quick calculation will show that very few of these can be stored on a standard 32-megabyte card, so you might want to invest in a larger storage card to take high-resolution pictures.

Professional photographers will argue that the best images are taken with a fixed focal-length lens. For close-up work, a lens that can take images at life size is best. This is called the reproduction ratio and life size is a reproduction ratio of 1:1. Thus a 35 mm slide of an object, say a paperclip, would have an image exactly the same size as the object itself.

You can tell what the reproduction ratio of your lens is using a simple test. Focus the lens as close as possible to a ruler showing a centimeter scale. With the ruler crisply in focus and as close as possible, the scale should read from zero to 35 mm. This is a reproduction ratio of 1:1 (Fig. 10.3). If the scale shows 70 mm the reproduction ratio is 1:2; 105 mm means a ratio of 1:3.

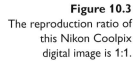

Figure 10.3
The reproduction ratio of this Nikon Coolpix digital image is 1:1.

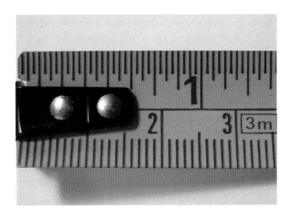

The quality of the lens is essential, so you should choose a respected manufacturer. It is still true that lenses for SLR cameras are generally better than lenses for digital cameras and as a result, image quality is easier to achieve. Experts will tell you that not only do you need a lens capable of a 1:1 reproduction ratio; you also need to have the correct focal length. For most images a 50 to 60 mm lens is used and for work at a longer distance, such as in the operating room, a 100 mm or even 200 mm lens is better. Most digital cameras have a 35 mm lens and this tends to distort the image, particularly the face, if used for close-up work.

A zoom lens is one way round this, allowing a variation in the focal length of the lens. Be aware also that electronic zoom is not true zoom and can lead to loss of image quality; it is the true zoom that you are interested in. Purists will tell you that the quality of images taken with a zoom lens is inferior to those with a fixed lens.

Furthermore, SLR lenses have a lower f-number, which is the factor for lens speed. Speed is nothing to do with how fast the lens moves. It refers to how much light the lens lets in through the aperture. By way of explanation, the lower the f-number, the better the light transmission. An f-2.8 lens will let more light in than an f-4 lens. This means that to achieve the same exposure, the f-2.8 lens uses a faster shutter speed, so the photographer is less likely to cause blurring due to camera shake. Zoom lenses tend to have a higher f-number than fixed lenses, so they need slower shutter speeds and are prone to camera shake.

Accurate focus is a problem in digital photography because the image is not seen through the lens and there is no guide to ensure accurate focus. Auto focus works well where there are crisp changes in tone but not where colors and tones are similar. This is particularly difficult with images of operations, where the tissues are tones of red. In addition, the lens will focus on an object in the center of the image, which might not be your area of interest. One trick is to set the camera to manual focus. The image is set-up and zoom and focus adjusted. You might find that temporarily placing a white ruler or similar object in the field allows crisp focusing. Now quickly ask an assistant to remove it before you take your picture.

You could take a series of images, gently moving slightly farther away and then closer, to ensure that at least some of them are in focus.

Flash is often useful but in most instances photographs should be taken in good ambient light. This is likely to create fewer shadows and better exposure. If in doubt, try both – after all, you can discard the worst images.

With most digital cameras the flash is fixed just above the lens. This 'axial' lighting creates adequate illumination in most cases. Professional photographers prefer to set the flash off from the axis of the lens to reduce red-eye, to enhance shadow detail, and to improve contrast. Unless the digital camera has a hot-shoe, this is not easy, although slave flash units can be used. Flat lighting using lighting from both sides and or a ring flash unit is beyond the scope of most (but not all) digital cameras. It does produce accurate color reproduction. It is also ideal for illuminating cavities.

If you work in an environment where you plan to take a lot of images, you might want to modify the environment to enhance photography. For before-and-after head and neck images, it is best to photograph against a matt white background. This can be achieved by fixing a board to the back of the consulting room door, or ensuring that a white wall is kept clean and free of clutter. White is preferable because you can use it to set your white point, to ensure that minor lighting variations are corrected, and, if you print images, it will save ink because white is not printed.

Alternatively, black or dark blue make excellent background colors; yellow and red should be avoided because they tend to dominate the image. For images to be comparable, you must use the same lighting, patient positioning, make-up, and camera distance/zoom. You can mark the floor for the camera distance. It is easy to make a cosmetic operation look better just by altering the lighting, make-up, and head position! If you use flash for the 'before' image, you must use it for the 'after' image as well. There is no place for trickery in showing the quality of surgery. A quick scan of many cosmetic surgery websites shows that this is common practice!

Readers interested in finding out more about correct positioning and exposure should read the *Handbook of Medical Photography* (see Bibliography for publication details), which includes very detailed information on taking standardized clinical images.

Reducing background clutter

Try to avoid all clutter around the subject – no instruments, wooden doors, posters, or additional personnel unless they are an essential part of the image. Any clothing that interferes with the shot should be removed and hair tied back. Jewelry and make up should usually be avoided.

Head and neck images

Standard head and neck images should be taken keeping the patient's Frankfort plane (a horizontal line drawn from the external auditory canal to the infra-orbital rim) parallel to the ground. This prevents a 'chin up' or 'chin down' view. The standard views that are recommended are summarized in the Westminster reproduction ratios.

If using flash, shadow in frontal views is restricted to those areas behind the ears and hair. If this is a problem, slave flash units on either side can be set up at minimal cost. These are driven by the camera flash and reduce or eliminate shadow (Fig. 10.4).

Figure 10.4
Good head and neck portraits
need careful lighting. This
image shows Dr Joe Niamtu,
who provided expert advice
on this chapter!

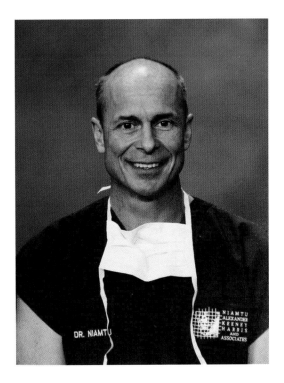

Oblique facial views are difficult to illuminate with flash. The nose and cheeks tend to cast strong shadows. A reflector sheet could be tried. Alternatively, try turning the camera sideways with the flash on the side towards the tip of the patient's nose, rather than the ear. This will illuminate the area behind the prominences better. Best of all is to use only ambient light, or to use the fill-in flash feature available on most cameras. You will need to practice to get this just right but, once mastered, you can use the same technique over and over again. To obtain comparable sequential oblique images, mark a dot on the wall and ask the patient to look at it at each photographic session.

For the undersurface of the chin, the nares, and the inframammary region, holding the camera upside down so that the flash illuminates from below can help.

Red-eye is a major problem in flash photography. If flash cannot be avoided, the camera's red-eye reduction feature might help. Strong ambient lighting will reduce red-eye. As a last resort, red-eye can be removed in Photoshop Elements®.

Macro images

Macro images (extreme close-up) can be taken with standard digital cameras. In traditional macro photography, the photographer tried to place the camera as close as possible to the subject. However, with digital cameras it is better to move back somewhat (perhaps a foot or so) and use the zoom feature. This will flatten the image, loosing the apparent depth of field but for most images this does not matter. It does improve lighting by keeping the camera and photographer out of the way. If flash must be used, the flash will not work if the subject is too close – it will miss the area of interest.

Good macro images require careful focusing. That does not mean that all of the subject need necessarily be in focus, that is a matter of artistic judgment (Fig. 10.5).

Figure 10.5
Macro images do not always have to be in clear focus, that is a matter for the artist! (Photography by Royal College of Surgeons Photographic Studios.)

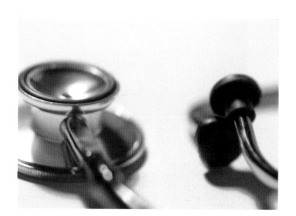

The operating room

Special considerations are needed for photography in the operating theatre. Natural light is less common in this environment but, if it is available, use it! In general, images should be taken with the operating light switched off, because this produces intense highlights that are too bright and leaves the periphery of the image in apparent total darkness.

Flash is difficult to use in this situation because the red color of tissue fools the flash, although a ring-flash if available works very well. Because slower exposures might be needed (which increase camera shake), you might want to consider using a tripod to support the camera if this is possible. Some theatres have a boom that you can fix a camera to.

You need to ensure that the viewers can orientate themselves, so take some images that show landmarks – the pelvis, the neck, anything that puts the image in perspective. Then focus down on the detail, keeping the same orientation, so as not to confuse the viewer. However, some images in the operating room are more photojournalism than anatomical record (Fig. 10.6).

You should try to get a 'surgeon's eye view', so politely displace the operator, stand on a high stool or step and take the image from above (Fig. 10.7). Do not fall into the wound – that might be the end of a glorious photographic career! Do not try to photograph over the surgeon's shoulder. This never works! As a general rule you should stand so that you get the camera directly above the incision. This usually means that the surgeon must stand aside. Politely explain why this needs to be; after all, he or she will want copies of the images, so it is in their interest to get the best shot. If you are not sure what the surgeon wants from the image – ask!

It is harder to avoid distractions in the operating room. It is worth taking time to surround the wound with fresh drapes (green or blue). Take out all possible instruments, although retractors may be needed to achieve the best view. Beware of reflection off metal retractors.

Figure 10.6
Images in the operating room can come in many guises (photography by Royal College of Surgeons Photographic Studios).

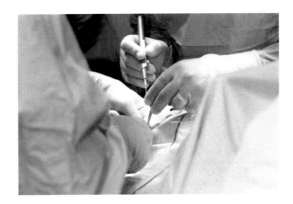

Figure 10.7
You should try to get a 'surgeon's eye view'.

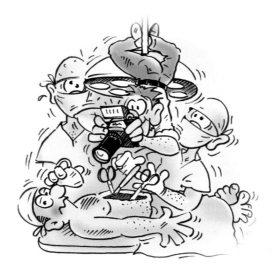

Remove lap pads (swabs) and get the lead for the bovie (diathermy) and the suction out of shot. Before doing so, use them to ensure a dry operative field. We usually irrigate with saline to clean up the field. Get the surgical team to change or at least clean their gloves. It might be worth asking them to hold a drape behind the operating table to provide a clean background. If not, make sure everyone is out of shot unless you feel they add to the image.

Despite our advice to remove as much clutter as possible, you might want to place a scale in the operative field. A simple white ruler will do well. This provides a sense of dimension.

If you are taking a series of images to illustrate how a procedure is done, be sure to take them all from the same place, with the same zoom and lighting conditions.

Pathology specimens

In the photography of surgical specimens, conventional 35 mm photography is gradually being replaced by image-acquisition systems that can quickly digitize an image, allowing far greater ease of use and integration into pathology and multimedia systems.

Figure 10.8
This high quality image was taken using the Argos™ system.

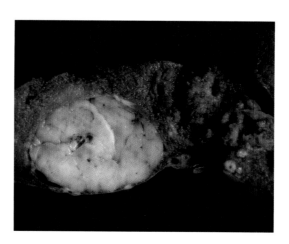

For example, the Argos™ digital imaging system, and the more advanced touch-screen version called Macropath™, are both macro (gross specimen) image-acquisition systems developed for the grossing and autopsy rooms (Fig. 10.8). Images are captured in 2 seconds and automatically digitally stored in universally accepted formats such as JPEG and TIFF, on a central server.

Through the local intranet the images can be readily accessed in the microscopy reporting room using a simple viewer program supplied with each unit, allowing the basic functions to assist in the reporting of routine histological specimens. The images are automatically retrieved, based on patient identifier number (including bar-code), allowing the pathologist to commence reporting with the benefit of simultaneous on-screen macro images with specimen measurements, site, and identifier of labeled representative blocks taken and microscopy slides. The ability to match the patient request form, macro images, and slides enhances quality assurance and eliminates the likelihood of errors. The systems can be set-up with the camera mounted on a wall bracket, within a fume-hood, or as a stand-alone unit on a wheeled trolley.

Pathvision™ is a dedicated image-management system developed to retrieve and manage images that have been acquired with Argos™ and Macropath™. It has the ability to recall their measurement calibration, allowing additional measurements in the microscopy room. In addition to many editing capabilities, the system allows additional image acquisition from other input sources, such as scanner, microscope-mounted digital camera, and video camera. This system enables the user to create a complete image profile of the patient for documents and specimen, which can be used as a teaching and research tool. The editing features of the software allow enhancement of images for publication and conference presentations, with features such as arrows, line drawing, text, and many other useful tools. An added feature is the ability to easily select and e-mail images in instances where a second opinion from a colleague might be required.

If such a system is available, use it! If not, try to reproduce the concept. Find a well-lit space, usually on the floor of the sluice! Lay the specimen flat on a clean towel or drape and place the camera directly above it. Use a large f-number (smaller aperture) if you can control this and – ideally – fix the camera on a tripod.

Skin lesions

Photographing skin is particularly difficult. You must try to reproduce the correct tones and focus must be crisp. If possible, place the area to be imaged on a firm surface so that at least only one of you is shaking! This is easy with arms and legs. For the torso or abdomen, the subject should lie down. Pay attention to lighting and focus using the rules above. Natural lighting is ideal, so move close to a window.

Photojournalism and candid shots

Taking informal images can be both more interesting and more challenging than the more traditional types outlined above. There might not be the time to set up the shot just as you wish, but careful planning can more than compensate for this.

Once you have selected the area where you want to work, be sure to ask permission of all the staff and patients who might be in the shot(s). You should probably also discuss your plans with the senior staff or managers first. Look carefully at lighting conditions, traffic flow, and backgrounds before deciding from where to shoot.

Think about camera settings if you can control these. For example, blur the background by using a shallow depth of field (by setting a small aperture). Consider whether to stand back and zoom in to allow the action to proceed as if you were not present.

The great advantage of digital imaging is that you can take as many images as you want and just keep the best ones. You can also learn about the composition as you go. Try bracketing exposures if your camera allows this, you might get dramatic effects.

Remember the rule of thirds. The image should have a focal point. Rather than placing this right in the middle, place it on a line one-third of the way from the top or bottom and one-third from the right or left border.

Try to tell a story. Look for interesting facial expressions: urgency, anxiety, elation.

Conclusion

After all this, we have one simple piece of advice. If at all possible, get a professional photographer to take your images! You will get much better quality images, consistent results, and, as you build rapport with your photographic colleague, you will both learn from each other.

Finally, if you are going to take your own images, be sure to carry consent forms with you. Someone might allow you to take a candid shot but unless you get permission in writing, the image cannot be used again. What a waste!

Bibliography

Stack LB, Storrow AB, Morris MA, Patton DR (eds) 2001 Handbook of medical photography. Hanley and Belfus, Philadelphia, Inc.

Chapter 11

Scanning images and X-rays

Terry Irwin and Julie Terberg

If you are serious about using images in presentations you should consider buying a scanner. We realize that not everyone needs or can afford a scanner, so in this chapter you will also learn how to get digital images of X-rays, transparencies, and other objects without a scanner.

If you want to scan your old 35 mm slides, you will need either a dedicated film scanner or a transparency adapter for a flat-bed scanner. Realistically, unless you are going to do a lot of scanning, you would be better off getting your best 35 mm slides scanned professionally – most high-street camera shops will do this (at a price). Once your whole collection is scanned and saved to a CD you can forget about slides forever!

If you want to scan images, such as pictures from a book, you will need a flat-bed scanner. If you are planning to scan X-rays, you will need a special type of flat-bed scanner that provides light from above the X-ray – a transparency scanner. Be sure to buy one that has a large enough plate to accommodate a full size X-ray. If you are a radiologist or do a lot of teaching using X-rays, it will be worth investing in a transparency scanner, but for most people there are ways to get around this problem that will do. Of course, if you are lucky enough to work in a hospital with a digital system, the radiology department will output image files on disk for you. You can learn how to do this in the next chapter.

For most of us, the best buy is a flat-bed scanner. These are useful for documents, images from books, and even solid objects. The image shown in Figure 11.1 was scanned using a relatively cheap Epson scanner. The image isn't on the real PDA, it was added as an extra layer (you will learn how to do that in Chapter 19).

A word of warning if you are considering buying a scanner: the resolution of the scanner will be described as 'interpolated' or 'optical'. Optical resolution is the true resolution. You will remember that interpolation is a software technique to fill in the gaps between pixels by guessing what color they should be. It is not a true reflection of the capabilities of the scanner.

Of course, a flat-bed scanner is much more than just an image input device. Modern optical character recognition (OCR) software allows the computer to recognize the text on the page and reproduces it in a word

Figure 11.1
A flat-bed scanner can be used to scan solid objects as well as documents (photography by Royal College of Surgeons Photographic Studios).

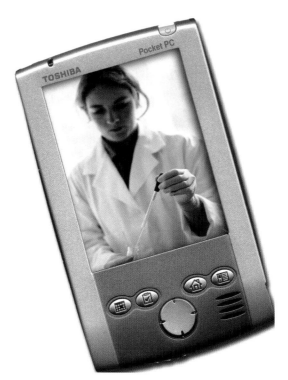

processing program. The scanner might also come with software to archive the scanned files. One of the best of these is PaperPort from ScanSoft, but there are many more.

Before we can discuss how to scan images and X-rays, we need to consider how a scanner works.

How scanners work

Most flat bed scanners are TWAIN compliant; what on earth does this acronym mean? Well in this case, actually nothing! It is said to stand for 'technology without an interesting name!' What it really means is that it is compatible with almost all image manipulation software, and in particular Adobe Photoshop Elements®.

The image or object to be scanned is placed on the top of the glass plate on the scanner. The lid is usually shut; leaving it open results in a black background. When the software on your computer tells the scanner to start scanning, the first thing that happens is that the lamp warms up. This can take several moments. The scanner then moves underneath and parallel to the glass plate and pre-scans the object.

As it does so, a light also tracks under the glass plate to illuminate the object. The reflected image is collected and redirected by a prism, which sends it to a charge-coupled device (CCD) – exactly the same as that in a digital camera. The digital signal from the CCD is sent to the software for image acquisition.

Figure 11.2
The opening splash screen in Photoshop Elements version 2 allows a shortcut to acquiring images from a scanner.

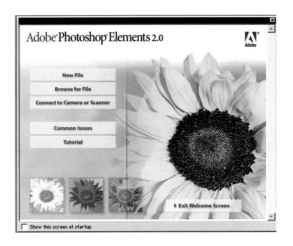

Figure 11.3
TWAIN settings on a standard flat-bed scanner.

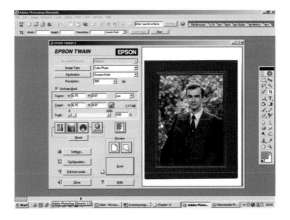

Scanning using Photoshop Elements

Place an object on the glass plate of your scanner, open Photoshop Elements and select 'Connect to Camera or Scanner' (Fig. 11.2). In Photoshop Elements version 1, the choice is 'Acquire'. If this is not visible, use the command File > Import > TWAIN.

Next choose a TWAIN source. Usually you will have only one – your scanner. However, if you have a video camera (web cam) or some other input device, this might show up. You will now find that the scanner pre-scans the glass plate and you acquire an image (Fig. 11.3).

Image type

To the left of the scanned image there are a series of choices. We need to go through each of the settings so that you can choose the optimum settings for your scan.

There are six possible types of image. These are 'Color Photo', 'Color Document', 'Black and White Photo', 'Black and White Document', 'Illustration', and 'Text/Line Art'. These are fairly obvious but what difference do they make? Although it is tempting to ignore them, don't!

The settings 'Color Photo' and 'Color Document' scan the object by recording the primary colors (red, green, and blue) for each pixel of the

Figure 11.4
Top left, color photo
(2.4 megabytes); top middle,
color document
(2.4 megabytes); top right,
black and white photo
(833 kilobytes); bottom left,
black and white document
(833 kilobytes); bottom middle,
illustration (264 kilobytes);
bottom right, text/line art
(20 kilobytes).

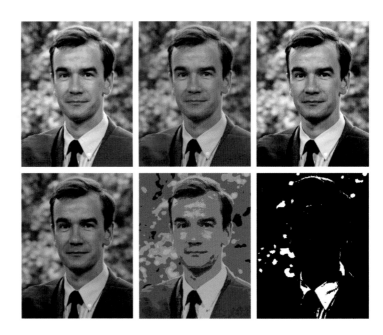

image using 1 byte for each channel (8 bits for each, so a 24-bit image). This will be three times the size of a black and white image, which scans using 1 byte for each pixel (8 bit image). So, if you are scanning a black and white image, or if you are scanning a color image but want to save it as a black and white image, choosing 'Black and White Photo' or 'Black and White Document' will reduce the file size to one-third of the size of a color image.

The difference with 'Document' (whether color or black and white) has nothing to do with bit depth (8 or 24) but with something called 'de-screening'. When an image is printed and then scanned (from a book, for example) the resulting image will have a moiré pattern. This is a curious herringbone-like pattern that results from the printed image. This is removed by de-screening. You can do this manually by scanning at very high resolution, blurring the image just a little and then sharpening it again using 'Unsharp Mask', but Photoshop does this for you, so why bother?

In the scanner setting 'Illustration', color smoothing is activated. Simply put, this reduces the number of colors that the scanner detects in an image and is applicable to images that are going to become GIFs (only 256 colors).

The images in Figure 11.4 were scanned at a resolution of 300 dpi, except the bottom middle and bottom right, which were set at 'Illustration' and 'Line Art', and scanned at 96 dpi. You can see that for this particular image, scanning as either a black and white photo or document results in the smallest image without loss of quality. The line art setting is the smallest file size, but quite unsuitable for this continuous tone image.

Destination

The TWAIN software likes to know what the image will be used for. If you open this dialogue box, the choices are self-explanatory. In reality, all that these choices do is change the resolution to suit the device that will be used to view the image (the output device). So for use on the web or on a screen, image resolution is set to 96 dpi, the maximum resolution of a computer screen. For printing it is set to a resolution appropriate to your printer and so on.

Resolution

You can choose the scan resolution yourself. If you are planning to enlarge your image you will want to scan at a higher resolution than the program will recommend. This is particularly applicable to 35 mm color slides.

Unsharp Mask

The Unsharp Mask filter should usually be ticked. It sharpens the final image (scanners tend to produce a rather soft looking image). This is particularly important with X-rays.

Source

You can ignore the source settings. When the TWAIN device has pre-scanned the page you will have a cross-hair on the screen. If you do not want to scan the whole page, click and hold-down the left mouse button to draw a rectangle around the area that you are interested in. The 'source' settings will change as you do this. They just describe the coordinates of the area that will be acquired when you scan.

Scale

This slider allows you to tell the scanner to enlarge your image. This can be useful when scanning color slides, so that the resulting image is larger than the original, but be careful not to enlarge too much. Most people prefer to scan at high resolution and enlarge with their image manipulation program (such as Photoshop Elements).

Auto-locate

This button, a white rectangle with a green rectangle within it, automatically selects the edges of the area to be scanned. You can try it to see if it works, but it is not always reliable.

Tools buttons

Three 'tools' buttons and an 'auto' button allow advanced users to adjust the appearance of the scanned image at acquisition. Just leave these as they are. The image is better scanned and saved first and then these adjustments made in Photoshop Elements, so that they can be undone if they do not work as expected. If you do change the settings, use 'Reset' to undo this.

Preview

Under the word 'Preview' there are two buttons. The left one scans the whole glass plate and the right one scans only the area outlined with the dotted box. When you have pre-scanned your object, select the area of interest with the cross-hairs; holding down the left mouse button while drawing a rectangle around the area of interest. You can adjust the boundaries after the box has been drawn, so don't worry if you are a little inaccurate.

Now click the right preview button to see a magnified view of the area of interest. Any fine-tuning can then be done before you make your actual scan.

Scanning in preview is much faster, especially if you are planning to scan at high resolutions.

Scan

The scan button then scans whichever area is selected. Depending on the resolution selected and the area to be scanned, this can take several minutes.

Settings

You really do not need to change any of the settings, alter the configuration, or use full auto mode (except if you are just scanning a full page). Don't forget the help button!

Choosing the correct resolution

This is the point at which you need to sit back and consider carefully why you are scanning the image. Let's assume that you have a 6 × 4 inch photograph that you want to scan and place in a PowerPoint® slide. If you scan at 100 dpi the image will be 6 (inches) times 100 (dots per inch) = 600 pixels across its long axis. If you are using a 17-inch monitor this will have about 1000 pixels across the horizontal axis, so the image will take almost two-thirds of the width of the monitor.

If you want the image to fill the slide area you should aim for a horizontal dimension of 700–1000 pixels (depending on how you have set up page size in PowerPoint), so scan at a slightly higher resolution. This way when you resize the image you can still have a high quality image at 96 dpi, which is the resolution of the majority of projectors.

When you are scanning to print an image, these constraints do not apply. The weakest link in the chain is no longer the rather limited resolution of your monitor but the print resolution. If you have a high-resolution printer such as a photo printer, you can scan at sufficient resolution to get high-quality images. This might be between 600 and 2400 dpi. Of course, the file sizes will be huge. A 6 × 4 inch photograph scanned at 100 dpi will be about 700 kilobytes, whereas at 600 dpi it will be 25 megabytes. If you are scanning images to be printed in a book or journal, consult the publisher's guidelines for optimum resolution. The images in this book are mostly at 300 dpi.

The scanner will scan the image to a file that has the same physical dimensions as your original, so a 6 × 4 inch photograph will produce an image that is 6 × 4 inches. Indeed, TIFF and JPEG files store this information in the file, although a GIF file does not. If you want to change the image size before printing, do this in Photoshop Elements but remember that if you want to enlarge the image, scan at higher resolution or you will lose quality.

Scanning an X-ray

You cannot scan an X-ray on a standard flat-bed scanner in the same way as you would scan a photograph or page of text. You need to illuminate the X-ray from above. You might be lucky enough to have access to a dedicated transparency scanner. If not, this section will help you overcome this. Even if

Figure 11.5
A CT scan image taken with
a 2.1-megapixel digital
camera hand-held in front
of an X-ray box.

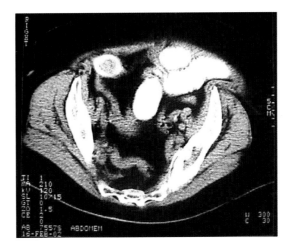

you have no scanner at all you can still get an image of the X-ray using your digital camera.

If you do not have access to a scanner, place the X-ray on a well-lit light box. Carefully align your digital camera with the X-ray. Even though it is hard on batteries, it helps to have the preview screen on the camera switched on. Look carefully at the resulting image. You will often find that there is a line representing the fluorescent tube. By carefully repositioning the camera, you can align the camera to eradicate this artifact, but it does take practice.

The CT scan showing a gallstone obstructing the terminal ileum was taken using this technique (Fig. 11.5). Images taken this way are certainly of good enough quality for use on the web or in PowerPoint. They might not be good enough to print in a journal or textbook, although this one was!

Once the images have been acquired, download them to your computer and open them in Photoshop Elements. Remember that your camera has taken color images and you only need black and white, so crop the images and convert them to black and white as you learned earlier. This will reduce the file size considerably. Now save them as a TIFF (which supports layers and does not reduce image quality).

If you have an ordinary flat-bed scanner there are two tricks that are worth considering. If you have access to an X-ray light box, place the X-ray on the scanner glass in the usual way. Now lay the light box on top of it and scan as usual. Alternatively, place two desk lamps, one at each end of the scanner and shine them on the X-ray. These techniques require a little practice and experimentation but with time you will obtain good quality images.

Scanning 35 mm slides

At the start of this chapter we suggested that if you had a collection of 35 mm slides you might find it easiest to take them to a high-quality photography store and arrange for them to be scanned for you. This is expensive but you need only do it once to preserve your valuable slides on CD forever.

When you buy a flat-bed scanner, you can choose to include the option of a transparency scanner and most of these have a holder for 35 mm slides. Before you insert the slide, make sure it is clean and free of dust.

Orientate it correctly. Scan at a high resolution (between 300 and 600 dpi) because you will want to enlarge the image later. The file size will not be huge because you are scanning such a small area.

It is even possible to scan 35 mm slides by placing them in a holder in front of a digital camera and taking images against a well lit background, such as a lamp or even a clear bright sky.

Conclusions

No matter whether you have the latest flat-bed scanner or just a simple digital camera, you should be able to obtain good-quality images of X-rays and 35 mm slides. Remember to save these as a TIFF file and to convert radiographs to black and white images to reduce file size.

By thinking about the purpose for which you are scanning, file size can be dramatically reduced so that your presentation will run smoothly.

Chapter 12

Digital radiological images

Terry Irwin, Bob Zeman and John Winder

Radiology encompasses a wide range of imaging techniques, from conventional X-rays through computerized tomography (CT), nuclear medicine, and ultrasound to magnetic resonance imaging (MRI). In the past, the most common medium for display and distribution of radiological images was acetate-based film. In general, only one copy of a film was available at any one time and in a single place. In some cases, a film had been lost and the radiological examination had to be repeated and photographed again.

Conventional radiological images are the equivalent of conventional photographic film. To convert these images to digital format they need to be scanned using a transparency scanner (also known as a film digitizer), or photographed with a digital camera (as described in Chapter 11).

It is interesting to note that digital radiological images have been with us for a long time in the form of CT, nuclear medicine, and – more recently – MR images.

These systems all required a computer for data acquisition and image reconstruction techniques. It was normal to acquire a high-quality image with these modalities and then print out on a film at much smaller size than the original screen display. We are reaching the stage where most radiological modalities are becoming digital, including ultrasound, computed radiography (CR), direct digital radiography (DDR), and digital mammography (which has been around for a long time). Modern computer systems are necessary to acquire, display, store, and transport radiological images. Access to and distribution of images will be via picture archive and communication systems (PACS) within a hospital and by teleradiology between hospitals. Images will be available at multiple places at the same time, at anytime, and at home. This also means that images are potentially available for teaching and inclusion in presentations in digital format, without the need for a scanner.

Older teleradiology systems use modem-to-modem connections over standard telephone lines (plain old telephone system; POTS) but more recent systems use some form of secure internet access using cable or DSL connectivity. T1 lines can also be used if high volumes of data are to be sent between institutions on a regular basis. Hospitals and medical offices within several hundred feet have also been successfully connected using wireless communication taking advantage of the 802.11b standard.

With the exception of analog, acetate-based films, radiological images have certain characteristics in common. The image is constructed from some form of measurement, it is processed for optimal presentation, it can be analyzed, and it can be stored in digital format or printed on a radiological laser printer. It is easy to scan the hard-copy output of such studies but this is tedious; it is better to access the digital information directly.

Modern radiology suites are fully digitized. Digital systems can capture twice the information of conventional systems because the data does not have to pass through a conventional analog image intensifier. The many other advantages of digital systems include the ability to enhance images, to link them to electronic patient information, and the transmission of images in real time to other areas of the hospital or beyond (teleradiology). However, although important, such issues do not concern us here.

Although not strictly the remit of this chapter, we feel that to understand the nature of the digital information, it will help readers to have some understanding of how modern radiological images are acquired.

CT combines a high-powered X-ray tube with solid-state or ceramic detectors. Most modern scanners are helical scanners, i.e. data is acquired during a continuous exposure made during one or two breath holds. As the patient is advanced through the gantry in one continuous motion, a volume of information is obtained along a helical path. Multiple slices of information are then reconstructed at predetermined intervals. In a single slice or single detector scanner, the sections that are obtained can be reconstructed retrospectively at closer intervals, or even with overlap. Their inherent thickness or collimation cannot be changed after the scan has been completed. Multislice or multidetector helical or spiral CT scanners allow multiple simultaneous sections to be obtained along parallel helical paths. This allows dramatically faster scan acquisition and enables the data to be reconstructed with thick or thin collimation, even after the scan has been completed. This major breakthrough allows very small lesions, which previously might not have been seen because of volume averaging, to be visualized and characterized. These CT slices can be used to reconstruct three-dimensional volume rendered views of the body. These three-dimensional images add a definite 'wow-factor' to a presentation (Fig. 12.1)!

Furthermore, advanced computer reconstructions enable radiologists to perform complex reconstructions, the cutting edge of which is exemplified by virtual colonoscopy.

MRI does not rely on transmitted X-ray. The subject is placed in a magnetic field 30 000 times stronger than the earth's static magnetic field. The patient's hydrogen nuclei, which have odd numbers of protons, align themselves with the magnetic field. A radiofrequency pulse is applied and switched off, exciting the protons to alter their orientation and spin characteristics; as they return to their baseline state they emit a radiofrequency signal that is detected by an RF coil, like a television aerial.

Nuclear medicine is over 50 years old. Sometimes unfairly referred to as 'unclear medicine', it involves the administration of specific radioactive isotopes, which accumulate in areas of the body. The faint gamma rays that they give off are detected by a gamma camera. If necessary, these signals can

Figure 12.1
Modern CT workstations can produce stunning three-dimensional studies.

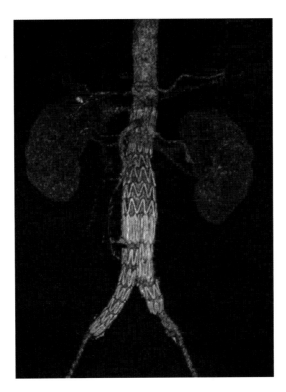

be color-coded to give additional information about signal strength and distribution in the body.

Although the spatial resolution of nuclear medicine is not as great as that of CT, ultrasound scanning (US), or MRI, it is a truly functional study that reflects as much about metabolic activity as anatomic structure.

Some nuclear medicine is performed using single photon emission computed tomography (SPECT). This technique uses rotation of the camera around the patient to produce three-dimensional tomograms that are typically displayed as axial, sagittal, and coronal sections. The images from these can also be saved in video (often as Audio Video Interleaves (AVIs)) or CINE format for later viewing as a rotating model. Thus videos of these studies can be exported directly to PowerPoint®. SPECT images can also be volume rendered, resulting in three-dimensional reconstructions of solid organs such as the heart. SPECT images will often show smaller abnormalities or very faint areas of uptake not evident on planar images.

A particularly exciting recent advance in nuclear medicine is the arrival of PET-CT. This combines modern helical CT imaging with positron emission tomography (PET). In a typical study, the uptake of fluorodeoxy glucose (FDG) is used to detect areas of increased metabolic activity. Malignant tissue typically shows greater FDG uptake than normal or inflammatory tissue. Electronic fusion of PET with the helical CT data allows precise anatomic localization of metabolically active neoplastic foci. Historically normal structures such as the neck muscles used to make the interpretation of PET difficult and resulted in reduced specificity. Refinements in technique, and the use of fused images, have dramatically changed this. In the future, no modern cancer center will be able to function without PET-CT.

DICOM image format

DICOM stands for digital imaging and communications in medicine. DICOM is a standard for the communication of medical images and associated information. In basic terms, the standard defines how medical images should be stored on a computer, transmitted between computers, and displayed on a computer screen. Each manufacturer must place patient details, scan parameters, and so on, in exactly the same place in the computer file so that other suppliers can view the image and the associated data. This allows the exchange of images between different systems from different manufacturers. It also defines the information needed to print images. Within radiology, nuclear medicine has been the last to implement DICOM, but even newer PET scanners are now DICOM conformant. Non-radiology vendors (such as those for cardiology) are also embracing the standard.

The official website on the development of this standard can be found at http://www.medical.nema.org/, but be warned; the DICOM standard is comprehensive! The DICOM standard has been in existence for some time and all major suppliers of radiological equipment conform to it, more or less. This has made the display and transfer of digital images easier and means that just one software package is required to display images from any modality. A very useful DICOM image viewer, called OSIRIS, can be found at http://www.expasy.org/www/UIN/html1/projects/osiris/osiris.html. It is free and relatively straightforward to use, allowing you to convert DICOM images into another format.

In practical terms, this means that any DICOM-based radiological study can be viewed on a PC that has a DICOM viewer. Although most DICOM viewers can handle traditional JPEG compression, some might have difficulty with wavelet or other advanced or proprietary compression schemes.

PACS

Picture archiving and communications system (PACS) is an image-based information system for the acquisition, storage, communication, archiving, display, and manipulation of medical images via the hospital network. PACS provides information to multiple users at the same time regardless of their location.

A further development of PACS is to design the system on a regional basis whereby a number of hospitals share the same database, enabling access to patient data from remote sites.

Most PACS systems can export images for use in PowerPoint, even removing patient identifiers in the process. Because the method of doing this varies from system to system, you will need to consult your local expert.

Although radiological workstations allow the operator to scan up and down, or indeed in any plane, through the images as if looking at a video, this cannot be exported readily. To reproduce this effect the images have to be exported to image manipulation software and an AVI made of the image collection.

Extracting digital radiological images

At present there is a wide age-range of radiological equipment in a modern hospital. Within the same department there might be a 20-year-old standard

X-ray system producing film-based images and multislice CT scanner producing only digital images. There might also be a range of different suppliers of equipment, each of which could differ in its method of image storage, archive devices (magnetic tape, floppy disk, optical disk, CD-ROM), computer operating systems (UNIX, LINUX, IRIX, VMS, MS Windows®), and networking methods.

Because of the range of storage media, network connections, and file formats, extracting radiological digital images from imaging systems has been problematic. For instance, an optical disk-drive that reads images from one manufacturer will be unlikely to read any other optical disks. A high degree of computer knowledge, cooperation from the equipment suppliers (who were often not very willing to allow hospitals access to their equipment's operating system), and an in-depth knowledge of image file formats was required to decipher or extract the medical image data.

The difficulty with accessing radiological images has begun to change with the advent of the DICOM standard. Most radiology devices now save images to media that can be read by PCs (such as CD-ROM) but better still is to send DICOM data to your computer (assuming you are on the same network) or access images through your radiology department's secure website (assuming they have one).

Computer files for storing radiological images vary greatly (for instance one could store 20 nuclear medicine images on a 3.5" floppy disk whereas it would take six 3.5" floppy disks to store one chest CR image). This reflects the fact that each imaging system will have its own image matrix size (pixels) and might require 1, 2, or 4 bytes to store each pixel. Sending images over your hospital's network is the best way to move this data around but should you have to use 'sneaker-net' instead, you will need media that has the appropriate capacity. Figure 12.2 shows typical image sizes (in megabytes) for some common radiological modalities. Note that these figures apply only to a single image from each machine and require to be multiplied by the number of images in an examination to determine the overall size.

Figure 12.2
Image sizes in radiology.

Imaging system	Single image size/Mbytes
•Digital subtraction angiography (DSA)	0.26
•Magnetic resonance (MR)	0.13
•Computed tomography (CT)	0.50
•Ultrasound (US)	0.31
•Computed radiography (CR)	8.00
•Nuclear medicine (NM)	0.03

Image transfer from a workstation in radiology

If you don't have access to a range of optical disk drives to read archived images from the optical disks then the best option is to network a DICOM-enabled PC to the imaging modality. Most radiology departments have such systems but you will have to ask a member of the technical staff to help you.

Most radiology devices support DICOM-send, that is, they can send to your networked PC. Whereas modern equipment also supports DICOM-query (i.e. you peering into their database and pulling a study), most vendors and radiology departments are unlikely to give you that access directly to the equipment. The exception is if they have an image server or web-server that is at arm's length from the radiologic system itself. If this is the case, they might give you query capability.

A number of products are available for use on PC systems to enable the user to receive DICOM images. The images can be displayed as thumbnails and written onto the local system's hard disk under a directory created by the software. The format of the images will be that defined by the DICOM standard and will range from approximately 100 kilobytes to a few megabytes depending on the image type and matrix size as explained above. Once the image is on your hard drive it can be viewed using a DICOM viewer such as OSIRIS and saved in a non-DICOM format for future use and insertion into PowerPoint or graphics programs such as Adobe Photoshop®.

Conversion from DICOM to formats such as bitmap, TIFF, or JPEG will save you a considerable amount of space on your hard drive. If you save the images in .DCM format they will be viewable only by DICOM viewers. This can be useful if it is necessary to retain demographics and scan parameters, but the file sizes are quite large. It is important to note that a CD writer, USB drive, or zip drive is essential if you are to get the images onto another PC, regardless of the format selected.

If you cannot receive transmitted images or load a DICOM viewer such as OSIRIS, visit the radiology department and (with permission) use their workstation, which will be equipped with a DICOM viewer. The system should allow you to save images to a zip disk or burn a CD in DICOM or graphics format.

If all else fails you might have to 'grab' the screen image and save it to disk. Press the 'Print-Screen' button on your keyboard to save whatever is currently displayed on the PC screen into the clipboard memory. This image can then be pasted into a graphics-editing program like Windows 'Paint' or, preferably, Adobe Photoshop Elements, where the relevant part of the screen can be cropped and saved. A useful tip if several windows are open is to hold down 'Alt' at the same time as you type 'Print-Screen' to capture only the active window, rather than the whole screen.

Using OSIRIS

OSIRIS is easy to master. You can download the latest OSIRIS viewer from http://www.expasy.org/www/UIN/html1/projects/osiris/osiris.html. We have placed a copy of version 4.18 on the CD with permission. Open the zip file and install it on your PC.

Now open OSIRIS (Start > All programs > Osiris4) and then open the file '_RGB.pap' by clicking on the file name and then choosing 'OK' in each dialogue box. Click the small video button to view the image sequence. Now choose File > Save AVI and select a frame rate of 12 frames per second. Save the file to your work folder.

You have now converted a set of DICOM standard images to an AVI file. When you have read Chapter 7 on inserting video into PowerPoint, you might want to try inserting this video into your presentation. Indeed, having learned how easy this really is, why not ask your radiologist to save a copy of an image or study for your next PowerPoint presentation!

Now open the 'Wrist.pap' file in OSIRIS (Fig. 12.3). Click Display > Invert colors to change to a positive image.

Figure 12.3
A DICOM image shown using OSIRIS (courtesy of Digital Imaging Unit, University Hospitals of Geneva, Switzerland).

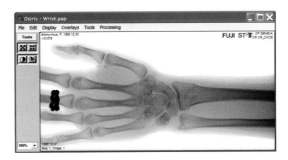

Choose Tools > Magnifying glass. Hold the cursor over the scaphoid bone and depress and hold the left mouse button. Here is the really tricky bit! Keeping the left mouse button depressed, click 'Alt' and 'PrintScreen' together. You can use your nose if you have short fingers! Now open Word or PowerPoint and click 'Ctrl V' or choose 'Paste.'

If you prefer, you can annotate the image using OSIRIS, although we recommend that you use PowerPoint for this. Choose Tools > Annotations and place the cursor where you want to type. Highlight the word 'annotation' and type your own text. The settings menu lets you change the font detail.

Future developments in radiology

In the not too distant future, radiology departments will cease to rely on acetate films and become largely dependent on computer-based display and transfer of images. PACS is composed of a central database, image review stations, short-term storage, a long-term archive, and a network infrastructure. A recently developed component of this is the radiology web server. There might be a number of these distributed on a hospital network and they will enable authorized users to utilize their office PC to access radiological images using standard web browser software.

Once acquired, radiological images will be stored centrally for reporting. Reported images will be sent to a web server for general access. It is very likely that some form of image compression ('lossless' JPEG or 'lossy' wavelet) will be employed for fast transfer of images around the hospital network. The degree of compression is controllable and will depend on factors such as network bandwidth and image type. Too much image compression will result in artifacts appearing in the images and not enough compression will result in slower image transfer times and impact on other network users.

Three-dimensional imaging will help enhance our understanding of pathology and injury. Many radiology vendors are already suggesting that, in future, images could be displayed initially as three-dimensional models, with the radiologist deciding where and how to slice the data after the fact.

Figure 12.4
A three-dimensional rendering of a pelvis produced using Three-dimensional doctor software (courtesy of Digital Imaging Unit, University Hospitals of Geneva, Switzerland).

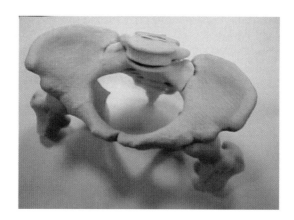

Figure 12.5
A three-dimensional rendering of the skull produced using Kismet software (reproduced by permission (origin: Forschungszentrum Karlsruhe http://www-kismet.iai.fzk.de/#TOP)).

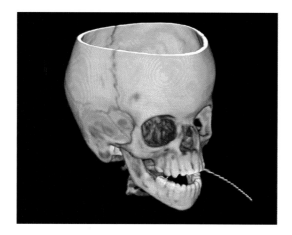

Some excellent examples of three-dimensional imaging systems can be found on the internet. Three-dimensional doctor (http://www.ablesw.com/3d-doctor/) is approved for medical imaging and uses vector-based tools to construct stunning images. The reconstruction of the pelvis shown in Figure 12.4 was produced using Three-dimensional doctor and is reproduced with permission.

Kismet uses specialized three-dimensional rendering and texturing techniques for volume reconstructions (Fig. 12.5).

In future digital image environments, accessing radiological images will be very much simpler, with users able to save individual images in a variety of file formats directly to their office PC.

Chapter 13

Saving and archiving images

Terry Irwin and Joe Niamtu

Most of us wish that we were more organized than we really are! If you are a keen teacher you will probably have amassed a substantial collection of images. The best doctors take a lot of pictures!

Some readers will have a large collection of 35 mm slides. These can be divided into three groups: clinical images, text-based slides and combinations of both. If you are 'going digital', the obvious question is what to do about this collection. As suggested in Chapter 11, you could just scan all of your slides, but this will be expensive if you have a large collection. Most of your text-based slides will be out of date and it is better just to rewrite and update these presentations as you need them. If the number of images is small, by all means scan them.

Alternatively, why not plan to replace all your images with higher-quality digital versions, using a decent digital camera. You do not need to do this all in one fell swoop. You can plan to do it as the opportunity and need arises. If you are speaking on a subject in the coming few weeks, think which images you need, plan to take them if the correct circumstances allow and then discard the old slides. If you cannot get the images you need, scan your old slides, but you might want to start a 'wish list' of images that you need for future reference.

It takes just a few seconds to capture an image of your routine cases, especially a picture that shows good anatomy or is in some way significant. Remember that common things are what we commonly teach about; rare cases are not always the best subject media. We often take images of procedures when we do not need them immediately. By doing this, a few images at a time, one can amass an archive of pictures.

No matter what your choice, you will need to save your precious digital files carefully. They can be stored in different directories on a PC, on CDs, on back-up disks or tapes, on external drives, and even on several different machines. Some authors advocate storing all of your images on the laptop that you use to give your presentations. This is a good strategy, especially if you have a CD burner, because you can carry all of your presentations and images wherever you go. That last minute change to a talk will be easy. You can work on the plane or train on your way to the meeting.

However, laptops are easily lost or stolen, so you must have a back-up strategy that ensures that you have the relevant files in your possession – and not in the same bag as the laptop! You will also need a full back-up of all your files at home or in the office.

When you go looking for images, you might wander aimlessly through these files or search your hard drive(s) using the built-in Windows® search button. Both methods are inefficient and can be extremely time consuming, although you might stumble across a long-forgotten image (this will happen some time after you really needed it).

You also need to consider how long you intend to store the images. We know that photographic film, if stored in the correct conditions, will retain its quality for many years, even several centuries. We cannot be certain how well CDs will last but it seems unlikely to be as long; it is uncertain whether they will last a professional career. Electronic files stored on computer seem relatively stable but we cannot be sure that they will outlive our needs. Nor are most of us happy that computers are inherently stable!

Some institutions that are building historic archives for the benefit of future generations take high-quality 35 mm or large-format emulsion-based images, scan these to electronic format and store the originals in ideal conditions. The quality of the electronic images will be superior to those taken with a standard digital camera, although the file size will increase as well.

For the majority of users, careful storage and back-up of digital files on a stable external hard disk drive is the next best and most practical solution. Do not store valuable images only on your main PC; if it crashes you will lose everything. External hard disk drives are now very reasonably priced and transfer of files using USB 2 (up to 480 megabits per second) or Firewire™ (up to 400 megabits per second) connections is very fast compared to traditional USB, which can transfer information at only 12 megabits per second (Fig. 13.1).

You should always establish a robust back-up strategy. This message is always best remembered after you have suffered a catastrophic loss of data! Modern external hard drives can store several hundred gigabytes of data for a fraction of the cost of the PC itself. This might be the best investment you ever make! The drives usually come with software that will automatically back-up your valuable files while you are asleep and/or at the touch of a button on the drive. If not, you should invest in back-up software.

To find the image that you need, when you need it, you require an image database. There are several excellent programs on the market. You can download trial versions of most of these programs and use them for

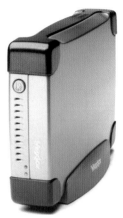

Figure 13.1   A Maxtor external hard drive. This drive holds 200 GBytes of data, more than most PCs. Transfer speeds are much faster than to CD or floppy disk, reaching 480 Megabits per second (image courtesy of Maxtor).

Figure 13.2
'This disk seems to be corrupted, would you like to try it in your PC?'

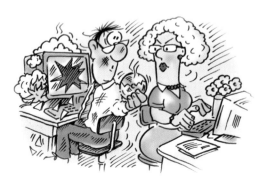

30 days. We have based this book on Adobe Photoshop® Elements because it offers excellent value for money and a user-friendly interface. Adobe has recently released Photoshop Album. This is a companion product to Elements and will meet most people's archiving needs. Alternatively, we have found ACDSee™ to be an excellent product, worthy of recommendation. There are many other similar products and ultimately you must decide which best meets your needs.

Using Photoshop Album

You can download a trial version of Photoshop Album from Adobe and archive up to 250 images without having to pay. If you are not familiar with this sort of program, this is a good way to see if it suits your needs. Go to http://www.adobe.com/products/photoshopalbum/download.html to get the software.

When you open the program for the first time you will be prompted to search your drive for images. This process takes a few minutes and images are then displayed in a slide sorter called the image well. A timeline along the top of the display shows when images were added (Fig. 13.3).

Figure 13.3
The Adobe Photoshop
Album workspace.

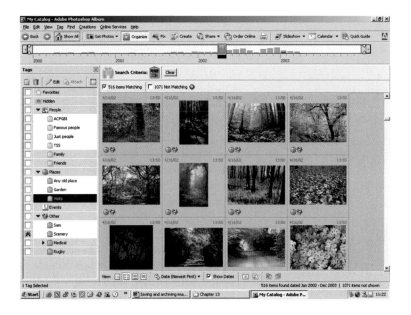

You can then work through the images deleting those you do not need. The program offers a choice; you can delete the image from the archive, or from the hard drive as well. Once you have selected which images to keep on your computer and which to store in your archive, you can add tags to the images. These are like luggage tags. You can select your own tags, either as categories or subcategories. For example, you might have the category 'radiology' and subcategories 'CT', 'MR', and 'other'.

Now go through the images in the image well and drag a tag to each image. You might want to associate several tags with one image. For example, an early cancer could fall under 'cancer' and 'pathology'.

You can also add information in the properties box. In particular, a caption is useful because if you display the image on a contact sheet or calendar this will be displayed with the image (Fig. 13.4).

Figure 13.4
The search pane in Photoshop Album showing all images with the tag 'pathology'.

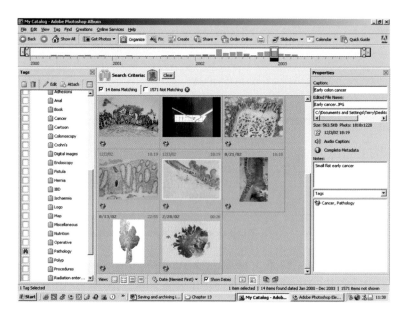

Once all of your existing images are in the archive you add further images using the program's 'Get Images' command.

Photoshop Album has simple search functions. Just drag the tag that you are interested in to the search bar or click on the box to its left. All the images with that tag will be displayed.

From time to time you might forget to tag images but Photoshop Album can easily search for these too, using the Find > Untagged Items command. The images can be tagged a number of ways; the simplest way is to drag the relevant tags onto the images.

Images that you use frequently can be tagged as 'favorites' and will tend to appear first in searches. You can also attach a 'hidden' tag, which will hide a rarely used image from searches until the hidden tag search box is displayed as well as your chosen search tag.

Backing up your images in Photoshop Album is very simple. The Backup command makes a copy of the catalogue and the photos, plus any video clips and audio clips you've brought into Photoshop Album, along with the folder structure they're stored in. You can back-up the catalogue to a hard drive or other media, such as writable CDs and DVDs.

Choose File > backup from the menu bar. Select the media on which you want to back-up the catalog; select 'Burn onto a CD or DVD Disc' to back-up to a writable CD or DVD. Select 'Specify Backup Drive' and then choose an external drive if this is your preferred choice.

You can create a full back-up to make a copy of the entire catalogue or you can perform an incremental backup to make a copy of the catalogue itself and recently added or modified images. Click 'OK'.

If you're performing an incremental back-up, insert the media containing the last full back-up and then follow the on-screen instructions.

Using ACDSee

ACDSee is part of a suite of programs for image manipulation, archiving, and storage. The features are broadly similar to Photoshop Album, although the interface is rather different. The images are displayed as slides, with a large version of the image available as well if desired. You can download the software from http://www.acdsystems.com; following the 'More' button will let you download a trial version.

ACDSee displays most of the functions as tabs for ease of use. It uses the familiar Windows file structure to find images. Images can also be stored in albums in the same way Photoshop Album uses tags (Fig. 13.5).

You can save information about an image directly in Windows XP when ACDSee is installed. Right-click on the image and select 'Properties'. The 'Image Properties' dialogue box will open (Fig. 13.6).

Choose the tab 'Database' and a dialogue box that allows you to add a description of the image, the date it was modified or added (defaults to today), the name of the author, and some notes and keywords will be displayed. When you subsequently open the image in ACDSee, these data will be displayed. This works either way round, you can add the data from ACDSee or through the Properties dialogue.

To use these programs to their full potential you do need to establish some discipline. You will need to take time to archive all of your existing images correctly, keeping them in designated folders. You will then have to add tags to the images using either of these programs. If you want, you can add brief descriptions of each image. This is laborious if you have a large number of images but it only needs to be done once.

Figure 13.5
Viewing images in a folder using ACDSee.

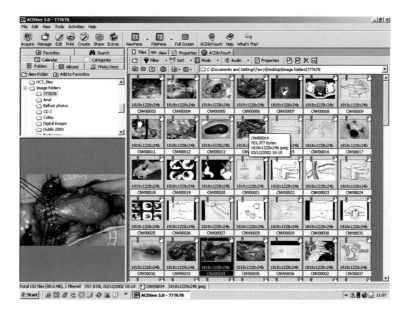

Figure 13.6
The properties dialogue
box in ACDSee.

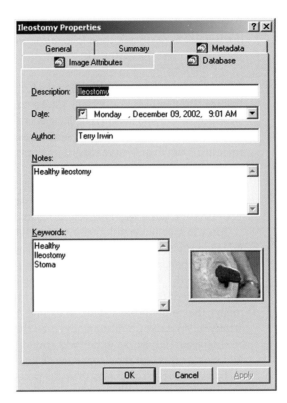

Using either of these programs you will soon have your image archive in good shape. Over the next few months you will build a superb database of images with clear information about each one and future searches will be quick and rewarding.

| Chapter 14 | # Image manipulation in Photoshop® Elements |

Image manipulation in Photoshop® Elements

Julie Terberg

To get the best out of your 35 mm images you could take them to a professional laboratory for processing and printing; for most people this is too expensive or complicated. Now, with Photoshop® Elements, you can perform many of the tasks of a professional laboratory on your desktop. Don't be inhibited by this, it is not as difficult as you might think. With practice, you can improve most images. Of course, because you will always make your changes to a duplicate, you will have the original image should you run in to problems.

The secret is to play around with the program to see what effects you can achieve. With experience you will get better at correcting common problems. If you are interested in learning more than is covered in this chapter, there are a number of magazines devoted to digital photography. These usually contain advice, tutorials, and even sample images to manipulate.

Image size and resolution

Earlier chapters have dealt with the importance of image size and resolution, so we can skip rapidly through this. We cannot emphasize enough the importance of safely storing and archiving your original image files before you start to alter them. These files will be huge but do not be tempted to compress them or reduce the resolution unless you are certain that they will be used only for purposes in which this is appropriate (on a PC or on the web). If you anticipate printing images, keep the originals.

To use an image in PowerPoint® or on the web, you must first determine the correct image dimensions. The table in Figure 14.1 is a suggested guide.

Figure 14.1
Suggested image dimensions.

Purpose	Horizontal image dimension	Resolution
Filling a complete PowerPoint slide with no border	800 – 1024 pixels (Depending on display setting)	72 – 96 dpi
Occupying a central portion of a PowerPoint slide	600 pixels	72 – 96 dpi
Set beside a column of text in PowerPoint	200 – 400 pixels	72 – 96 dpi
As a logo in the corner of a PowerPoint slide	75 – 100 pixels	72 – 96 dpi
On the web	100 – 400 pixels	72 dpi
On an A4 sheet for printing, occupying ¼ page or less	1750 pixels	300 dpi or the maximum resolution of your printer
A full A4 sheet (landscape)	3508 pixels	300 dpi or the maximum resolution of your printer

To change the size of an image, open the file in Photoshop Elements. Ensure that 'Constrain proportions' is ticked so that the vertical dimension is changed at the same percentage as the horizontal. Select Image > Resize > Image Size and retype the horizontal dimension. If necessary, edit the resolution. Click 'OK' and then select File > Save As, using a new name in an appropriate directory.

Cropping

If you crop images in PowerPoint, the cropped area disappears from the slide but the information is not deleted, so the file size remains the same. In PowerPoint 2002, you have the option to compress your images and delete the cropped areas, which will greatly reduce your file size. For the greatest control over your images, we recommend that you use Photoshop Elements for all editing purposes, including cropping.

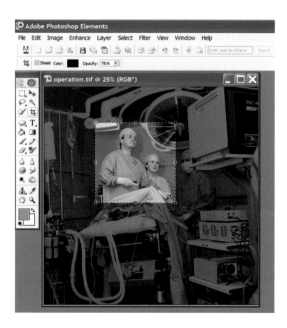

Cropping and straightening images

Figure 14.3   It is amazing how you can crop a single image to obtain several very good images (photography by Royal College of Surgeons Photographic Studios).

To crop an image, open it in Photoshop Elements and select the Crop Tool. To try this yourself, open the file 'operation.tif' from the chapter folder. Place your cursor towards the top left corner of the area that you want to crop, click the left mouse button and drag (hold button down) the selection box to the lower right corner of cropping area (Fig. 14.2). Release the mouse button.

You will notice eight squares ('handles') on the corners and sides of the selection box. Click and drag on any one of these handles to adjust the crop selection. You could also place your cursor inside the selected area and click and drag to move the entire selection box around your image. If you place the cursor just outside the handles, a small curved arrow will appear. Click and drag an arrow to rotate the crop selection. We demonstrated this in Chapter 3. You can crop multiple images from one original (Fig. 14.3).

There is a shortcut to straighten images in Photoshop Elements (Image > Rotate > Straighten Image) but this does not always produce the results you expect!

Correcting for perspective

When you take photographs of buildings, especially tall buildings, they will appear to narrow as they rise. This distortion can be corrected to achieve much more realistic-looking images.

Open the image 'buildings.tif' from the Chapter 14 folder using Photoshop Elements. Note how the buildings appear to narrow as they rise. Before making any transformations, you need to make the Background layer an editable layer. If the Layers palette is not visible, open it by selecting Window > Layers. Double-click 'Background' in the Layers palette to bring up the 'Layer Properties' dialogue box. Type in a new name for your layer, such as 'transform', and click 'OK'.

Select Image > Transform > Perspective. Note the eight handles that surround the image. Click on one of the top corner handles and drag it horizontally to change the perspective (Fig. 14.4). You can also skew the

Figure 14.4
Transform perspective: dragging the handles changes your image perspective (photography by Royal College of Surgeons Photographic Studios).

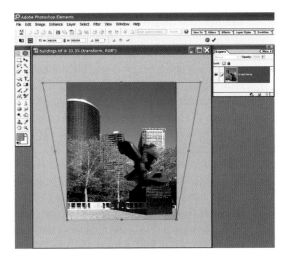

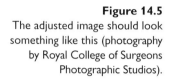

Figure 14.5
The adjusted image should look something like this (photography by Royal College of Surgeons Photographic Studios).

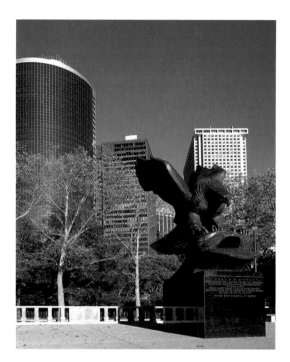

image by moving these handles up and down, but the effect is rather more abstract! Click the Move Tool (arrow icon, or any other tool) to apply your transformation (Fig. 14.5).

Color saturation

Healthcare professionals do not have the time, expertise, or facilities to arrange perfect lighting conditions for every image. As a result, skin tones can appear dull or pale, and artificial lighting can leave a color cast. It is possible to correct for these problems, although this takes considerable practice.

We are not going to go into detail about this, but will address some common issues. Open the image 'P-J.jpg' from the Chapter 14 folder on the CD. This is a very nice image showing the facial characteristics of Peutz-Jegher syndrome. However, the image shows rather flat skin tones. In Photoshop Elements, select Enhance > Adjust Brightness / Contrast > Levels.

You will see a graph depicting the saturation of each color. There is very little white in this image, so the graph has a long flat tail. Click the small arrow under the right side of the graph (not the lower slider) and drag it to the left. Notice how this improves contrast, particularly of the darker tones. Similarly, drag the left arrow to the right until you are happy with the result. At the top of the 'Levels' dialogue box, notice the box labeled 'Channel'. You can select and adjust each of the red, green, and blue channels separately (Fig. 14.6). This is useful if there is a color cast, perhaps from artificial lighting.

You can produce some interesting effects by converting one or two channels (red, green, or blue) to monochrome and leaving the third as it is. Select Enhance > Adjust Color > Hue/Saturation and choose one of the colors from the 'Edit' box at the top. When you drag the Saturation slider

Figure 14.6
Brightness levels: just by adjusting the sliders on the brightness level graph, the image contrast is dramatically improved.

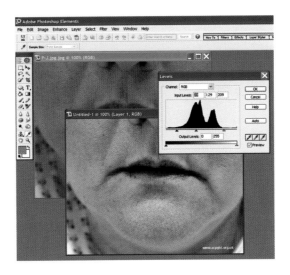

Figure 14.7
Hue/saturation: an image made more dramatic by highly saturating the yellow channel (photography by Royal College of Surgeons Photographic Studios).

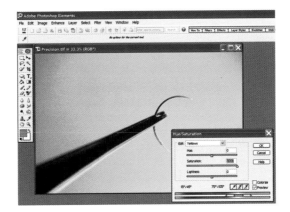

completely to the left, that color will be translated into gray values, or monochromatic. If you drag the Saturation slider to the right, that color will become more intense. Try this on the image 'precision.tif' from the chapter folder (Fig. 14.7).

Setting the black and white points

In Photoshop Elements there is a simple technique that will adjust tone and contrast and greatly improve the appearance of your images.

Select Enhance > Adjust Brightness/Contrast > Levels. You will see three small eyedroppers in the lower right corner of the dialogue box. The left dropper sets the black point. Click this and then click on a point in the image that is closest to pure black. Next, click the white dropper and choose the area that is closest to pure white. Do not select an area that is very overexposed. The final step is to select the gray point. Click the gray point dropper and choose an area of your image that is, as the name suggests, medium gray. Note how the use of these three droppers enhances the

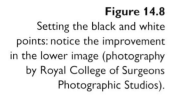

Figure 14.8
Setting the black and white points: notice the improvement in the lower image (photography by Royal College of Surgeons Photographic Studios).

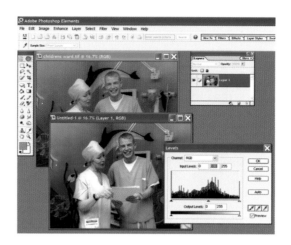

contrast and color depth. Almost all images will benefit from this treatment; try it on 'childrens ward.tif' if you like (Fig. 14.8).

Dodging and burning

More experienced users may want to darken (burn) or lighten (dodge) areas of the image. Remember to save your image first! A useful trick for editing is to make a copy of the image as a new layer. To do this, make sure that the Layers palette is open. If not, select Window > Layers. Now click on the thumbnail image in the Layers palette and drag it down to the copy icon, which looks like a page with the bottom left corner turned up. You can work on the copy layer rather than the original background. If you find that you've gone too far with your editing and want to start again, drag the copy layer to the trashcan icon in the lower right of the Layers palette. Select the Background layer and copy it again. When you are satisfied with the final image, delete the background layer by dragging it to the trashcan icon in the lower right of the layers palette.

Open the file 'Buildings.tif' and select File > Save As and give the file a new name such as 'burndodge.tif'. Using the Crop tool, select an area that contains the statue of the eagle. Apply the crop and select File > Save. With the Zoom tool selected, click on the 'Fit on Screen' button from the Options menu bar across the top.

The Dodge and Burn tools are located in the Toolbox menu on the left side of the screen (Fig. 14.9). These tools are based on traditional photography techniques for changing exposure on specific areas of a print. Use the Dodge tool to bring details out of shadowed areas and the Burn tool to bring details out of highlights.

Select the Dodge tool and adjust the size of your brush to about 100 pixels. Select the Midtones range and change the Exposure to about '35%.' In the shadowed areas of the statue, begin bringing out some of the detail. If you find that you've gone too light, you can always use 'Ctrl Z' or 'Undo' to go backwards and try again. It's important to keep the shadowed areas darker than the surfaces that the light is hitting, or your image will not appear realistic. Keep a light hand at this.

Figure 14.9
The Dodge tool and
the Burn tool.

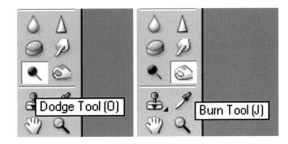

Figure 14.10
Dodge and Burn models:
notice the detail in the
shadowed areas.

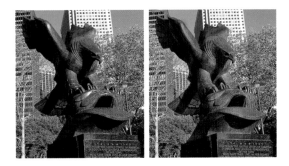

The Burn tool is located right next to Dodge in the Toolbox. Select this and adjust your brush to about '60 px', the range to 'Highlights', and the exposure to '30%'. Brush lightly in the strongly highlighted areas on the statue, pulling out a little more detail and slightly darkening the harsh highlights. Again, don't overdo it and keep your image realistic (Fig. 14.10).

Sharpen filter

Photoshop Elements offers at least 90 different filters, most of which offer various settings to customize your filter options. The best way to familiarize yourself with the filters is to experiment on different images and see what happens when applying different settings. We will cover a few of the filters and how you can use them to manipulate your images and make them more effective.

The Sharpen filters work by increasing the contrast of adjacent pixels, helping to improve blurred images. Open the file 'sharpen orig.jpg' from the chapter folder. With the Layers palette open, drag the Background layer to the copy icon to duplicate the layer for editing. Rename your new layer 'Sharpen'. Select Filter > Sharpen > Sharpen and take a look at the resulting image. Make another copy of your Background layer in the Layers palette, and try some of the other Sharpen filters (Fig. 14.11).

Figure 14.11
Left, original image; second from left, Sharpen Filter; middle, Sharpen More; second from right, Sharpen Edges; right, Unsharp Mask (photography by Royal College of Surgeons Photographic Studios).

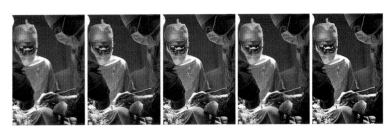

Blur filters

The Blur filters soften a selection or an image. Blur and Blur More have the least impact on an image, but still work by averaging pixels in contrasting areas. Gaussian Blur quickly blurs your image by an adjustable amount, typically producing a hazy effect. The Motion Blur filter has adjustments for direction and distance, similar to a moving object taken at a fixed exposure. Smart Blur precisely blurs an image based on the options of your choice.

The Radial Blur offers a couple of dramatic effects based on 'Spin' and 'Zoom' methods. You have a variety of settings to explore and you can also change the position of the Blur Center so that it begins on the focal point of the image.

Figure 14.12
Radial Blur filter: adjust the blur center (photography by Royal College of Surgeons Photographic Studios).

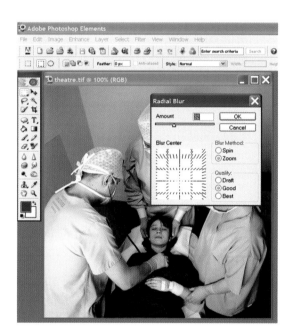

Figure 14.13
Example of Radial Blur Filter (photography by Royal College of Surgeons Photographic Studios).

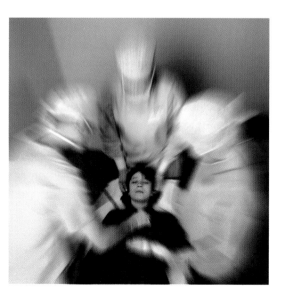

Open the file 'theatre.tif' and select Filter > Blur > Radial. Under Blur Method select 'Zoom', and under Quality select 'Good.' Adjust the amount slider to about '32' and drag the Blur Center to approximately the position of the patient's face. Click 'OK' to see the Radial Blur effect on the image. You might not be satisfied with the results and want to make some adjustments. Select Edit > Undo or 'Step Backward' (Ctrl Z) and then select Filter > Radial Blur and reposition the Center, or change the Blur 'Amount' (Figs 14.12 and 14.13).

Retouching specs, dirt, and other spots

Even with the utmost care, dust and dirt can work their way into your images. Lenses get dirty, and transparencies and scanners magnetically attract dust and hair. Fortunately, it's pretty simple to retouch your images in Photoshop Elements and get rid of any unwanted spots.

Open the file 'buildings.tif' and select the Zoom tool. Click and drag a box in the upper left corner of the image, concentrating mostly on the blue sky. The image should be at a zoom level of about '140%' or more, so you can easily see all of the dark spots in the sky.

Next, select the Clone Stamp tool from the tool menu on the lower left. You have many options on brush types and sizes, and opacity settings. The brush size can also be adjusted by using the left and right bracket keys on your keyboard '[ ]'. This makes it easier to scale your brush size as you're working. Move your brush outline in the blue-sky area, just to the right of a dust spot and holding the 'Alt' key down on your keyboard, click the left mouse button and then click again on the dust spot. This sets the origin point for your clone stamp, and now you can start 'stamping' on all of the dust spots. Each time you click the mouse, notice the cross hairs are oriented exactly the same as your first origin point. Any time you wish to grab a new origin point, just hold down the 'Alt' key and select the new position.

You can use the Clone Stamp tool to retouch a scratch in an old photograph or eliminate a telephone line across a skyline (Fig. 14.14).

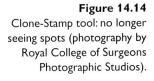

Figure 14.14
Clone-Stamp tool: no longer seeing spots (photography by Royal College of Surgeons Photographic Studios).

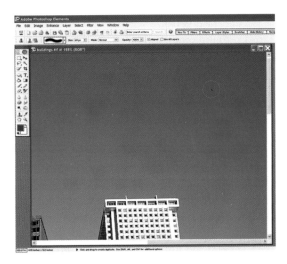

Erasing

The Eraser, Background Eraser and Magic Eraser allow you to erase areas of an image using transparency. One of the best ways to understand these tools is to apply them to an image. Open the file 'eraser orig.jpg' and make a copy of the Background layer in the Layers palette. Rename this layer 'effects layer.'

Select Filter > Blur > Radial Blur. Slide the amount to approximately '30%' and move the Blur Center to about the same position as the surgeon's fingers. Now you will use the Eraser tool to pull out some of the details of the instruments and the surgeon's hands, making these the focal point of your final image.

Select the Eraser tool from the Toolbox and set the brush for about '50 px' and the opacity at '50%'. Begin erasing the blur effects from the surgeon's fingers; keep erasing until you see all of the detail from the original. Change the brush size to about '80 px' and slide the opacity down to about '30%'. Use this eraser setting to pull out a little detail from the surgeon's face (Fig. 14.15).

Figure 14.15
Blur filter applied, Eraser brings back details (photography by Royal College of Surgeons Photographic Studios).

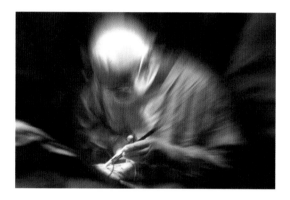

There are many uses for the Eraser tools. You can learn more about them, and their uses, in the Photoshop Elements Help file.

Selection tools

The first tool in the Toolbox is the Rectangular Marquee tool. This is just one of the ways you can select a smaller area of your image for editing. Other selection methods include the Lasso tools, the Magic Wand tool and the Selection Brush.

Quite often, you only want to edit a portion of your image, such as making the background area darker, or changing the color of a certain part of the image for highlighting. To select specific areas of your image, you need to become familiar with the Lasso tools. The Lasso and Polygonal Lasso tools allow you to select freeform or straight-edged areas. The Magnetic Lasso tool automatically snaps to the edges you cross over while selecting and is especially useful for selecting complex images from a high-contrast background.

For this example, open the file, 'lasso orig.jpg' and make a copy of the Background layer in the Layers palette. The objective of the exercise is to select the background area behind the two subjects and to darken this area to make the foreground the focal point of the image.

Select the Zoom tool and zoom in so you can see the details of the edges around the people. Select the Polygonal Lasso tool and begin clicking points around the top left edge of your image, continuing to trace points around all of the background area. If you want, select a small section and then add to this by using the 'Add to Selection' mode from the options menu bar at the top. Don't forget to select the small background area just underneath the man's face (Fig. 14.16).

Figure 14.16
Using the Lasso tool (photography by Royal College of Surgeons Photographic Studios).

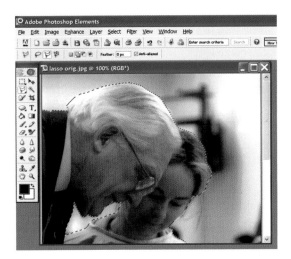

When you have finished selecting the background area, choose Select > Feather from the menu bar. Change the Feather Radius to '2 pixels' and click 'OK'. This will soften the edge of the selection area.

The next step is to darken the selected area. Select Enhance > Adjust Color > Hue/Saturation and drag the Lightness slider to '−60'. This amount can be adjusted however you like, and whatever works for your particular image. Click 'OK' and then Select > Deselect (Ctrl D) to view your adjusted image (Figs 14.17 and 14.18).

Another very useful selection tool is the Magic Wand tool, which allows you to select an area of similar colors without having to trace the outline. The Tolerance setting varies from 0 to 255. Use a lower setting to select colors that are very similar to the first pixel you click and use a higher setting for a broader range of colors in your selection.

Open the file 'buildings adjusted.jpg' and select the Magic Wand tool. Set the Tolerance to '44' and click anywhere in the blue sky. The selected area should include all of the blue sky. Let's add a slight blue gradient to this selection. Select the Eye-dropper tool from the lower portion of the Toolbox. Click anywhere near the bottom portion of the sky to change the foreground color to a light blue. Hold the 'Alt' key and click on a dark blue area of the building; this will change the background color to a darker blue. Next, select the Gradient tool from the Toolbox. The default gradient should be 'Foreground to Background'. If this is not the gradient that appears in the shaded box on the options menu, click on the gradient and select the first box under 'Presets' (Fig. 14.19). Click 'OK' to accept this preset. Now click near the lower portion of the sky on the buildings image and then drag the cursor up near the top of the sky and release the mouse button. The sky should appear darker at the top. Type 'Ctrl D' or choose Select > Deselect to view the new sky. Select File > Save As, and save your file with a new name.

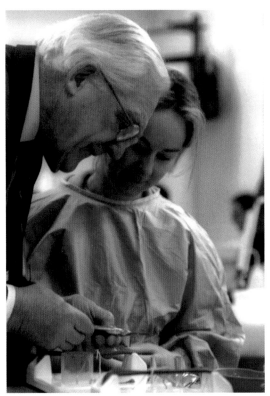

Figure 14.17 Original image (photography by Royal College of Surgeons Photographic Studios).

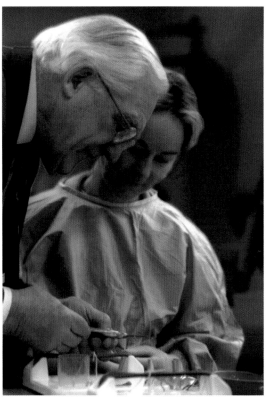

Figure 14.18 Lasso tool used to select background area for darkening (photography by Royal College of Surgeons Photographic Studios).

Figure 14.19 Using the Gradient tool presets (photography by Royal College of Surgeons Photographic Studios).

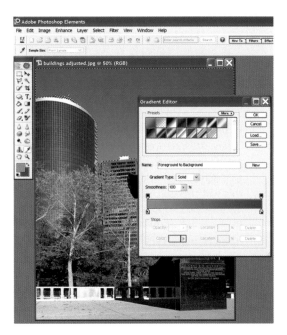

Adding text and arrows

Many medical images benefit from annotations with text, arrows, and color highlights but radiological images provide the best examples.

Open the image 'colon.jpg' from the Chapter 14 folder on the CD. We want to highlight the dilated transverse colon, the site of the obstructing sigmoid cancer, and the dilated small bowel. Begin in the Layers palette by making a copy of the Background layer. Select the Magic Wand tool and change the tolerance to '32'. Click inside the dilated transverse colon (the black bit at the top) to make your selection (Fig. 14.20).

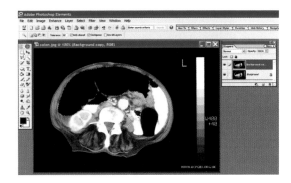

Figure 14.20
Using the Magic Wand tool to make a selection.

The next step is to soften the edge of your selection. Choose Select > Feather and change the Feather Radius to '2 pixels'. Click 'OK'.

To recolor your selection, select Enhance > Adjust Color > Hue/Saturation. Tick the box next to 'Colorize' in the lower right corner of this dialogue box. Move the Lightness slider to the left to approximately '+25'. Adjust the saturation to approximately '50' and then the hue to about '200' or any blue color (Fig. 14.21). Experiment with different hue/saturation settings to learn what this tool can do for you. Type 'Ctrl D' to deselect.

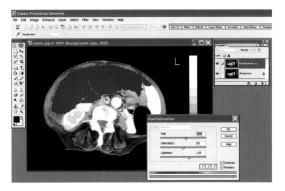

Figure 14.21
Enhance > Adjust Color > Hue/Saturation to 'Colorize' a selection.

The next step for this image is to highlight the region of the cancer. Because this area consists of many different values of gray pixels, the Magic Wand tool will not help us make our selection. Choose the Selection Brush tool from the Toolbox. Change the brush size to about '7 pixels' and start 'painting' on the area you wish to select.

Next, with your selected area still active, choose Enhance > Adjust Color > Hue/Saturation. Tick the box next to 'Colorize' in the lower right corner of this dialogue box. Then slide the Hue slider to about '40' and set the saturation to '70' (Fig. 14.22). You can adjust the Lightness slider for further enhancements. Click 'OK' when you are satisfied with the color.

Figure 14.22
The Selection Brush was used to select the area of the cancer, which was then colorized.

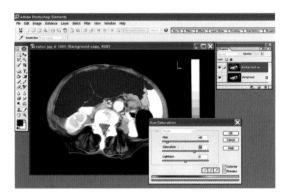

Now, we'll highlight the dilated small bowel. Again use the Selection Brush to highlight this area and adjust the hue and saturation to achieve a color that stands out. We used a feather setting of '2 pixels', colorized the image and set the hue to '0', saturation to '55', and lightness to '−10' (Fig. 14.23). Type 'Ctrl D' to deselect.

Figure 14.23
The small bowel was highlighted.

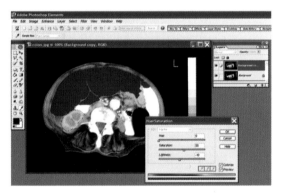

The next step for this image is to add text labels for each highlighted area. Select the Text tool and place the cursor over the transverse colon. Select 'Verdana' as your font, a point size of '24', and white or black, depending on which area you are typing into. You might want to add drop shadow from the layer styles menu. When finished typing, click the Move tool (arrow icon or 'Ctrl V') and place the text in its final position (Fig. 14.24).

Finally, simplify the image by merging all the layers. Before you do this, save a copy of the file as a .psd file so that you can come back and change the layers if you want. Now select Layer > Flatten Image and save your file as a TIFF.

Figure 14.24
The text labels were added.

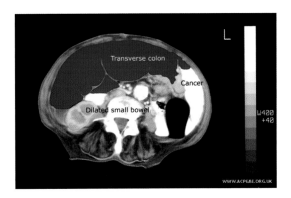

Chapter 15

Consent, ethics, and the law

Terry Irwin and Charles Oppenheim

Ten years ago it was accepted practice to take images of patient care without regard to consent, except perhaps where the patient was easily recognizable from the image. In the last decade doctors have recognized that patients are entitled to know that images have been taken and for what purpose. However, few healthcare staff have really considered the issue of consent in any detail. The situation is further complicated by data protection law in many countries (see below) and more recently by the Health Insurance Portability and Accountability Act (HIPAA) in the USA.

Basically, when a patient permits the recording of an image it cannot be assumed that this constitutes consent. The patient has a right to know what purpose the image will be used for, who will see it, whether it might be copied and or distributed, and for how long it will be available. It is also important to agree who will have access to or use the image. Will it be available to a limited number of local, professional educators or can anyone make use of it? It is also reasonable that the patient should know what efforts will be made to secure the image and thus prevent use outside the specific areas for which consent has been given.

It is not just patients who need to give consent. The image might include relatives, visitors, or staff, who might object to having their image included in the output. In addition, the image could contain equipment or facilities that are of a sensitive nature.

In considering these issues, we need to take each step in the image processing in turn. During this discussion the terms 'patient' and 'subject' are used synonymously, as are 'image' and 'recording'. We hope that those who refer to their charges by other terms, such as 'clients', will not be offended!

Taking the image

The question of consent must be considered before the image is taken if at all possible. There might be instances when an image is taken of an unconscious patient and the question of consent arises at a later time, but this should be exceptional. In the USA, filming patients for public viewing without consent in a place that they might expect to be private (e.g. an examination cubicle) is an unlawful violation of privacy[1–3].

Figure 15.1
Filming patients without consent in a place that patients might expect to be private, is an unlawful violation of privacy.

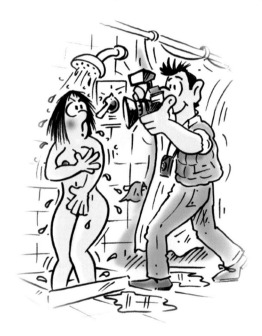

It is not clear whether the act of filming or just the broadcast/transmission of the image is unlawful, but in most countries it is considered unethical to film or broadcast without specific informed consent in advance.[1,4] The presence of a photographer who is not appropriately qualified might also be regarded as unethical.[3]

The act of taking the image must not allow the treatment of the patient to be delayed. Nor must it be assumed that a patient in an emergency situation (who might be in distress) can necessarily give valid, informed consent.[5] For these reasons, the American Medical Association specifically recommends that filming (the recommendations refer mainly to video) should be restricted to those patients who can give specific informed consent.[6] It would be ideal practice that consent be taken by a third party to avoid any conflict of interests.

The subject should be approached before preparation is made to take the image and given a clear explanation of the purpose and nature of the image. It is not good enough just to 'pop into the ward' and ask a patient to smile for the camera! A relative or other surrogate cannot give valid consent for photography except in the case of a minor. Where the subject is a minor or is incapable of giving consent because of mental incapacity, great care should be exercised. Although it is often regarded as acceptable to obtain consent from a relative, it would be unwise to obtain an image when it is clear that the patient is unhappy about this.

Patients might reasonably assume that the image is being taken either to monitor their progress or for teaching of staff. If it is your intention to use the image in a book, to publish it in a journal, to use it on the internet, or to use it in an advertisement, it is unethical not to say so and you will not have obtained proper consent.

There are some images for which consent is not necessary, although this varies from country to country. If in doubt, it is always best to err on the safe side and obtain consent. In the UK, these issues are overseen by the General Medical Council. The GMC suggest the following guidelines:[7]

- Seek permission to make the recording and get consent for any use or disclosure.
- Give patients adequate information about the purpose of the recording when seeking their permission.
- Ensure that patients are under no pressure to give their permission for the recording to be made.
- Stop the recording if the patient asks you to or if it is having an adverse effect on the consultation or treatment.
- Do not participate in any recording made against a patient's wishes.
- Ensure that the recording does not compromise patients' privacy and dignity.
- Do not use recordings for purposes outside the scope of the original consent for use without obtaining further consent.
- Make appropriate secure arrangements for storage of recordings.

There are circumstances when the GMC considers that consent is not mandatory:

- images taken from pathology slides
- X-rays
- laparoscopic images
- images of internal organs
- ultrasound images.

This does not preclude obtaining consent, but formal written consent is not required in such cases. It might still be good practice to seek verbal consent and to record this. Indeed, the GMC states that:

> Such recordings are unlikely to raise issues about autonomy and will not identify the patient. It may nonetheless be appropriate to explain to the patient, as part of the process of obtaining consent to the treatment or assessment procedure, that a recording will be made.

When a recording is made as part of the assessment of a patient, for example to document the progress with complex reconstructive surgery, it is not necessary to obtain written consent but it is wise to explain why the recording is being made and to record that verbal consent has been taken.

Your responsibilities do not end when an image or recording has been taken. It is wise to allow the subject to see the recording and to confirm that he or she is happy for it to be used for the intended purpose.[3] It has been established in law in the USA that the subject has the right to withdraw consent after images are taken[8] and this is certain to apply worldwide. In these circumstances the image must be destroyed and not simply archived.

There are particular rules for the recording of images at post-mortem (autopsy) and advice from the local coroner's office should be sought if there is any doubt.

What if the patient refuses?

If the subject declines to have images taken, you cannot proceed. If images have already been taken, they must be destroyed.

It is important to reassure patients that it is their right to decline to have images taken or to withdraw consent after the images have been taken and that this will not affect the quality of care that they receive.

If you have explanatory materials and/or a consent form, the patient must be given adequate time to read this and to consider their options.

Who should take the images?

It is essential that those who take images have a full understanding of their responsibility to protect patient confidentiality. Ideally, the individual should be a healthcare worker directly involved in the patient's care or a professional photographer employed specifically for this purpose, but if this is not possible, staff have a responsibility to ensure that the person(s) involved are aware of their duties and legal responsibilities.[6]

Using the images

Images should be used only for the purpose for which consent was obtained. If you want to use the images for any other purpose, you will need to seek further consent from the subject. Of course, if the patient is not recognizable from the image and/or they fall within the categories of image for which consent is not mandatory anyway, this will not be necessary.

The issue of whether the patient is identifiable is not always clear-cut. It is important to bear in mind that even when the patient's face is not visible, they may be recognizable from some other feature. They might have a distinctive tattoo or surface feature. In other cases a patient might recognize his or her own image and conceivably this could cause distress (say, for example, in the case of a limb amputated in an unusual form of accident). Indeed, the procedure that you are recording might, in itself, identify the subject. Again, the golden rule is always: if in doubt, get consent.

Images taken in exceptional circumstances

There might be circumstances when you feel that it is in the patient's interest to make a recording without consent, for example in cases of suspected non-accidental injury in children. Considerable caution should always be exercised in such cases. Junior staff should seek experienced counsel and not act on their own volition. The GMC provides useful advice for staff in the UK in cases of doubt.[7] This is similar to advice given in other countries but you are advised to check. Alternatively, it is wise to check with your protection society or insurer.

Financial benefit from taking of images

It would be unethical for healthcare staff to benefit financially from the taking of images (still or video) or their participation in filming of commercial material.[3] However, in the case of educational materials (such as this book), if the use of images is essential and the subjects are aware that the images will be used in this manner, or have assigned copyright to you, this is acceptable.

Storing the images

The images taken on a digital camera will usually be stored on removable media. It is important to remove them from the camera and save them safely on a computer as soon as possible. Digital cameras are easily stolen and you could lose more than a few images. If the patient's legal team seeks access to the images at a later date you will need to show that you took steps to ensure their protection.

You might be required to demonstrate the security of image storage in the UK[7] and in the USA.[6] This means that you have a responsibility to ensure that your computer is at all times physically secure (under lock and key if not in your immediate possession) and that data is protected by a secure password/encryption or both. You should install a firewall to protect your computer from unwelcome intrusion from hackers (a free firewall can be downloaded from www.zonealarm.com).

Although we have not explored regulations elsewhere in the world, it would be surprising if they were not similar.

Once safely transferred to a computer, the original images on the removable medium should be deleted. Remember that images on a laptop are just as susceptible to theft as images on a digital camera, and it too must be kept securely locked away at all times.

Images and video recordings can form part of the patient's medical records, even if taken for educational purposes. It is not clear whether in law they are discoverable either in the USA[6] or in the UK (personal communication: Medical Protection Society). Nor is it clear whether *all* images might be discoverable in law, or just those in which the patient is identifiable or for which he or she gave consent. In other words, the legal position with respect to an image of an operation is uncertain. This is an important issue, because any image that is discoverable needs to be archived in such a way that it can be retrieved, and thus it must be cross-referenced against the subject. In the UK this means that the database on which the images are stored must also be registered under the Data Protection Act.

There are a number of software programs for archiving images; indeed most digital cameras and scanners now provide such programs with the bundled software. You might therefore consider using one of the programs detailed in Chapter 13 and cross-referencing images against the patient identifier.

Video images must also be stored in a secure environment; this means behind lock and key.

Data protection law

Data protection laws exist in many countries, including all European Union (EU) member states. The USA does not have a Federal data protection law, but a number of Federal and State laws protect patient privacy to a greater or lesser extent. The recent Health Insurance Portability and Accountability Act has significant implications for protecting confidential patient information.

The account that follows refers to the law in the EU. Readers are strongly advised to refer to standard texts on the topic for the country in which they practice for further guidance. It should be stressed that this section of the chapter refers to legal factors that are applicable *in addition* to the general guidance provided in this chapter.

The basic principle of data protection legislation in the EU is more to do with good practice in handling personal data than to give a legal right to privacy. None the less, in practice, it does provide considerable protection for personal privacy. Data protection law applies to information about a living, identifiable individual. To fall under the ambit of the law, that information must be linked directly or indirectly to details about that individual, such as name and address. It makes no difference whether the information or data is computerized. Images of patients, as long as those patients can be readily identified, fall under the ambit of the law. In the EU, there are particularly stringent rules about so-called 'sensitive personal data'. This includes data about an individual's health or sex life. Images of a patient will generally fall under this heading.

In essence, it is an offence to 'process' (and this term includes making, manipulating, disclosing, storing, or merging) such sensitive personal data except under very restricted circumstances. One of these is to 'protect the vital interests of the data subject'; general opinion is that this refers to saving the life of the patient in an emergency and nothing more. Certainly, creating a PowerPoint® presentation including patient images would not count. A second (and in practice, the only realistic) circumstance is when the individual has given his or her explicit informed consent, that is, has given consent in writing and has had a full explanation of what might be done to the images, who might see them in future, how long they will be maintained, and so on. If patients are incapable of giving such informed consent, perhaps because they are children, or because of physical or mental incapacity, then explicit written permission must be sought from others, for example parents/guardians. If this is not possible, then no images should be made.

Data protection law also gives data subjects the right to be told if any data about them is being held, what that data is, where the data was obtained, and who has seen that data. They have the right to sue for damage (including distress) caused to them by any breach of the data protection law, or to demand that particular data be corrected or erased. All of this potentially applies to images of the patient intended for use in PowerPoint or similar presentation packages.

To assess whether the images in question are likely to be subject to data protection legislation, one must consider whether the patient is identifiable, either directly from the image alone or from the image in combination with other data held by the organization processing the data. It is likely that even when the image is apparently anonymous (e.g. shows a detail of the body without showing the patient's face or other characteristic feature), the patient can, in principle, be identified from other records in the organization (e.g. the date the picture was taken, linked to records of operations carried out on that day, linked to a database of patients due for operations that day). Readers are advised to exercise great caution, as Courts take into account the sensitivity of the data and the distress caused by unauthorized disclosure when deciding on damages and criminal penalties for those who breach the local data protection law. It should be noted that someone could sue to prevent disclosure of personal data that might cause the individual *or anyone else* (e.g. relatives) damage or distress.

It should, however, be noted that the law only applies to *living* individuals. Images taken of corpses are therefore not subject to the law, although the advice set out in the remainder of this chapter still applies.

It is also important to remember that it is a breach of the law to dispose of patient images in such a way that unauthorized third parties can see them. Thus, when disposing of obsolete computers that have been used to create PowerPoint presentations that include patient images, care must be taken to ensure that no third party can inspect the contents of the hard drive. Similarly, you should exercise great caution when disposing of CDs containing images or old PowerPoint presentations.

Existing images

Most healthcare professionals will have existing collections of images. In many cases, patients can be identified and it is true that in most instances written consent will not have been obtained for the use of these images. It is recommended that images that would now require consent are replaced with suitable alternatives wherever possible. Images that would not now require consent can still be used.

Images for use in journals

Most reputable journals will now insist that written consent for the use of all images is given before publication. Under no circumstances should images that are subject to data protection law be submitted without such explicit consent. Data protection law applies locally. Thus, for example, images that appear in a journal that is widely circulated in, say, the UK, might be subject to the UK Data Protection Act even though the images were originally created in another country.

Consent forms

Every hospital or practice will develop its own consent form or adopt one from an umbrella organization. Appendix 1 shows a consent form that is suitable for most purposes. This form is available on the CD accompanying this book and you are free to print and use it, but please acknowledge the source.

Processing non-digital images

Although this book is about digital imaging, not all images are in digital format. Some staff continue to use 35 mm film to obtain slides, color prints, or monochrome images. Some material used for promotional use will be obtained on large-format cameras.

It is all very well securing the patient's permission to take and use the images but a patient will be very upset to find that the film has been processed in a public place, without regard to security or confidentiality. This is particularly true of images of a sensitive nature.

Every hospital or practice must have robust protocols for handling traditional film; this will usually mean processing in-house.

Transmitting digital images

The widespread availability of e-mail in healthcare allows the rapid transmission of digital images. However, transmission of a digital file via e-mail risks potential access to the file by unauthorized computer users.

As an e-mail moves across the internet it is transmitted as a series of packets (clusters of data). These packets are transmitted from one node on the internet to another. The message can be intercepted at any of these nodes by a malicious hacker. The best way to protect images is to save them to disk and transport them personally, but if you must transmit them electronically they should be encrypted. This is no longer the stuff of spy films.[9] The most popular encryption algorithm is PGP.[10]

Editing images

Whether one is considering still or moving images, most will be edited before they are used. However, any image that is discoverable must be retained in its original format. That means that digital images must be saved full size and video must be unedited.

It is very unwise to offer 'souvenir copies' of video images to patients. However, if the patient requests copies of images, it is difficult to see how this can be refused.

Copyright and ownership

The ownership of images taken within healthcare institutions is a complex issue and to our knowledge has not been tested in law. In most – but not all – countries, copyright of an image taken by a member of staff as part of his or her employee duties belongs to the employer, not the member of staff. However, this simple statement covers many complex situations. You will have to establish what the law has to say about such issues in your own country, as copyright laws do vary a lot from country to country. Also, it is often not clear what the member of staff's employee duties are, although if one is a resident photographer paid to take images of patients, then the situation is clear. Other members of staff might have contracts of employment that are silent about taking images, or about copyright in general.

Even if in theory the legal position is clear, custom and practice might be quite different. For example, if medical staff are routinely allowed to do as they wish with text and images they create, then a Court might take the view that the employer has in effect waived its right to copyright. So, whereas it seems reasonable to regard any image taken on healthcare premises to be the property of the hospital or practice in whose jurisdiction it was taken, in practice the situation is not clear-cut. In particular, most staff taking images regard them as their own property. As the healthcare provider has legal responsibility for ensuring the safe-keeping of images, it seems possible that they are indeed also the owner of the images. This matter can cause tension. For example, when members of staff leave the employment of one healthcare organization and move to another, are they allowed to take copies of images with them?

This is a complex area where the law, custom and practice, and contracts of employment overlap, and legal or trade union advice might be required.

It is wise for each institution to develop written guidelines that cover this issue and make clear the obligations of staff. The institution should also make clear that publication of images without permission might not only be a breach of confidentiality but also a breach of its copyright.

However, there is little point in having such rules unless they are applied regularly. Turning a blind eye in the past will greatly weaken an employer's case in the future.

If images that are not owned by the employee or the employer are copied, for example from a book or from a web page, it is not invariably an infringement of copyright. Concepts such as 'fair use' in the USA, 'fair dealing' in the UK, and 'private copying' in much of Europe might apply. To avail oneself of such a defense, the person copying must demonstrate that the copying does not damage the legitimate economic interests of the copyright owner, and is for one of the permitted purposes allowed for in the particular national legislation. For example, in the USA, such permitted purposes include:

- criticism
- comment
- news stories
- teaching
- scholarship
- research.

In the EU, copying for research is restricted; only copying for non-commercial research (however that might be defined) is a permitted purpose.

When doing such copying, the user must consider four issues:

- The nature of the work being copied.
- The amount and substantiality of the portion copied ('substantiality' refers to the importance of the material being copied rather than its amount).
- The nature of the use (and, in particular, whether any commercial product will result).
- The economic impact on the copyright owner.

Together, these factors are weighed up to determine whether a particular use is fair.

Care must be exercised in copying and using material published on the worldwide web, including images. Unless specifically stated otherwise, material published on the web is normally protected by copyright law.[11] There is not necessarily any implied license to copy. If in doubt, seek permission from the copyright owner.

Many countries, especially those in the EU, also have laws of moral rights, which make it an offence to amend an image (e.g. by cropping) without the permission of the creator of that image, and which require the creator's name to be associated with the image.

Copyright is murky legal territory and the law is often counterintuitive! Readers are strongly advised to take legal advice when dealing with any third party materials or when negotiating with employers over what can be done with images they have taken.

Conclusion

In this chapter we have tried to explore the complex issues of consent, ethics and copyright. These are not simple issues and will require further reading.[12] It is preferable to avoid involvement in establishing case law, so our advice is simple:

- Always obtain informed written consent unless existing guidelines and laws specifically state that it is not necessary in your country.
- Save images securely as soon as possible in their unaltered, original format.
- Be aware of copyright law when reproducing others' images.

Appendix 1

Hospital name

Consent for medical photography, imaging of investigations or procedures

> Affix label or add name, date of birth,
> address and unit number

Please read this form very carefully. If there is anything that you do not understand, ask the staff who are looking after you to explain it. **You have the right to refuse to have images taken and this will not affect your treatment in any way**.

I consent to the recording of photographs and/or video recordings of me, my operation or procedure or my tests such as X-rays for the following purposes:

Please indicate each type of use to which you are happy to give consent by initialing in the right hand column	Initial here
As a record of my care or current clinical condition (that is to show how I look now or how I may have changed).	
For teaching, examination or other educational purposes. The images may be used to teach students or other doctors or nurses, both within the hospital and elsewhere. The images may be used in examinations to test students' or doctors' knowledge.	
For publication in printed materials such as medical or nursing journals, educational articles or booklets. These will be available to the public as well as other doctors and nurses.	
For reproduction on the hospital intranet (which means that staff of the hospital may see images from computer screens within the hospital but they cannot be seen by anyone outside the hospital).	
For publication for educational purposes on the internet (worldwide web) for educational purposes only. This means that other professionals and in some cases, members of the public may see the images and even copy them to their computer.	
Specifically, I consent to images being sent by email (electronic mail). This form of mail can be intercepted in transit by others who are intent on doing so, though this is rare.	

I understand that I can withdraw my consent at any time, even after the images have been taken. Of course if the images have been published in a book, journal or magazine it may not be possible to withdraw my consent. I understand that I may specify which of these purposes the images may be used for (by initialing only those I do wish to consent to).

Signed: _____   Date: _____

Witness: _____   Name of witness: _____

This form may only be witnessed by a doctor of Specialist Registrar grade or above or by a nurse of 'F' grade or above.

References

1. Green *v* Chicago Tribune Co, Illinois App. 1996 1st Dist. 1st Div.
2. Council on Ethical and Judicial Affairs, American Medical Association, Opinion 5.04. Communications media: standards of professional responsibility, in code of medical ethics. Current Opinions with Annotations, 2000. American Medical Association, Chicago.
3. American Medical Association. Filming patients in health care settings. Online. Available: http://www.ama-assn.org/ama/upload/mm/369/report_118.pdf (accessed April 2004).
4. Millar v National Broadcasting Corp 1986 Cal. App.
5. American College of Emergency Physicians, Ethics Committee 2001 Recorded images: use and abuse in the emergency department. Online. Available: http://www.saem.org/newsltr/2001/may.june/filmingp.htm (accessed April 2004).
6. Practice brief: patient photography, videotaping and other imaging (updated 2002). Online. Available: http://library.ahima.org/xpedio/groups/public/documents/ahima/pub_bok2_000585.html (accessed April 2004).
7. General Medical Council 2002 Making and using visual and audio recordings of patients. Online. Available: http://www.gmc-uk.org/standards/AUD_VID.HTM (accessed April 2004).
8. Virgil v Time Inc 1975 9th Circuit US App.
9. Julie Meloni. Encryption tutorial. Online. Available: http://hotwired.lycos.com/webmonkey/programming/php/tutorials/tutorial1.html (accessed April 2004).
10. PGP home page. Online. Available: http://www.pgp.com/index.php (accessed April 2004).
11. Brad Templeton. Ten big myths about copyright explained. Online. Available: http://www.templetons.com/brad/copymyths.html (accessed April 2004).
12. Oppenheim C 2001 The legal and regulatory environment for electronic information, 4th edn. Infonortics, Tetbury, Gloucestershire, UK.

Chapter 16

Typography

Julie Terberg and Terry Irwin

Just as this is not a PowerPoint® or Photoshop® Elements manual, it is most certainly not a manual of typography. However, some basic rules of typography are essential if your presentation is to be visually effective.

Modern typography began when Johannes Gutenberg and William Caxton developed mechanized systems for printing. The mirror image of individual letters were cast in lead and arranged in order, ready to be inked for printing. The spaces between lines were filled with lead strips, hence the term for the spacing of lines – leading (rhymes with heading). The letter was surrounded by a small amount of space to stop ink from connecting adjacent letters. Modern word processing is basically the same process; it is just a lot faster and easier. However, some things are possible on a computer that could not be achieved easily on a mechanical printing press.

We are no longer constrained by the 'bounding box' – the space surrounding each letter. It is possible to expand the space around letters or to overlap the spaces (condensing the text). We can also orient type vertically or at any angle, warp text for special effects, or even layer transparent text over other objects.

Fonts

We refer to the appearance of type as the 'font', from a French word for 'casting'. A font family can include a series of typeface variations such as normal, bold, italic, extended, thin, and so on. Today, the terms 'font' and 'typeface' tend to be used synonymously.

Until the 1980s only a limited number of fonts and font sizes were available. This changed when Adobe® introduced the PostScript® Type 1 system of fonts. These were derived from mathematical vector equations and could be scaled up and down in size without compromising the quality of each letterform. Each Type 1 font includes a screen font and a scalable printer font. Type 1 fonts are preferred by printers and print designers, and are well supported on the Mac platform.

147

Not wishing to be tied to a single company, Apple® and Microsoft® collaborated to develop the TrueType system of fonts. TrueType fonts are scalable and include all of the screen and printer information in one file.

Only TrueType or the newer Open Type fonts can be embedded with a PowerPoint presentation.

! ! ! ! ! ! ! ! ! ! ! ! ! ! ! ! ! Note !

Embedded fonts are fonts that are packaged along with your presentation file, so that when it is viewed on another system the text will appear exactly as intended, even if that system does not have the same font. With each installation of new software – Microsoft or otherwise – you will incorporate a new set of TrueType fonts in your fonts folder. Your font list is unique to your system and the programs that you have installed. It can be very difficult to determine whether the next system to display your presentation will include exactly the same font list.

You can select any TrueType font for use in your presentation. However, if you try to embed a font with a license restriction, a message will appear with a warning and you should make another font choice. To prevent last-minute problems, try embedding any unique fonts early on in your presentation development.

! ! ! ! ! ! ! ! ! ! ! ! ! ! ! ! ! Note !

To embed fonts with your PowerPoint 2000 file, select File > Save As > Tools > Embed TrueType Fonts. To embed fonts in PowerPoint 2002: select File > Save As > Tools > Save Options and select the appropriate option for your current document.

You do not have to embed the base fonts that come with Windows®, which are:

- Times New Roman
- Arial
- Symbol
- Courier New.

To determine if your font is TrueType, look for a small shadowed 'T' to the left of its name. In Figure 16.1, the first three fonts are TrueType and the two versions of Albertus are not. A statement will also appear at the bottom of the dialogue box confirming a TrueType font.

Figure 16.1
Font dialogue box.

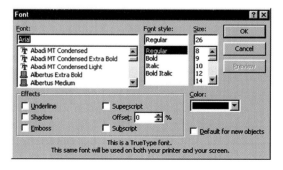

Point size

Type size is measured in points. A point is 0.0138 or 1/72 of an inch. Point size is supposed to represent the distance from the top of the ascender (letters such as b, d, and h) to the bottom of the descender (as in g, p, and q). This is only a guide, as different fonts of the same point size will not necessarily be identical in dimension because of variations in weight and design (Fig. 16.2).

Figure 16.2
Different font samples, same point sizes.

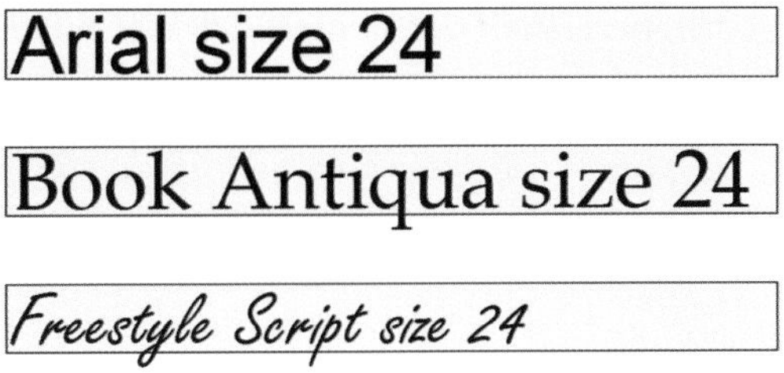

Arial size 24
Book Antiqua size 24
Freestyle Script size 24

Choosing the correct font

The reason for choosing a font depends on its purpose. Some fonts are best suited for large headlines or titles, others for smaller text. Some are purely decorative and designed to be eye catching and different. Also, it is important to recognize that typefaces have personality. Whether they seem traditional, modern, corporate, fun, shocking, subtle, or somewhere in between, the fonts you choose can communicate a feeling or mood to your audience.

Typefaces are categorized by appearance and can be divided into a few basic groups: serif, sans serif, script, symbol and decorative (or display).

Serif fonts

Serif fonts have flourishes, or extensions, off the main strokes of each character. These fonts are said to be easier to read in paragraph form when printed but the serifs tend to become blurry when viewed at small sizes on a monitor. Our recommendation is to use serif fonts sparingly in your presentations, limiting them to titles and larger headings or phrases.

!!!!!!!!!!!!!!!! Note !

One exception to this rule is Georgia, a serif font specifically designed for a 72-dpi monitor (Fig. 16.3).

Figure 16.3
Serif font examples.

Serif font examples
Times New Roman
Book Antiqua
Garamond
Georgia

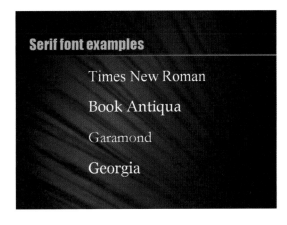

Sans serif fonts

Sans serif fonts (the French word 'sans' means 'without') are typefaces without serifs. They read well in most sizes and also when they are reversed (light text on a dark background). Their legibility makes sans serif fonts the best choice for presentations. Two sans serif fonts – Verdana and Tahoma – were specifically developed for use on screen (software and web applications). Both of these fonts were designed to be very legible at small sizes and they are supplied with newer versions of Microsoft Office (Fig. 16.4).

Figure 16.4
Sans serif font examples.

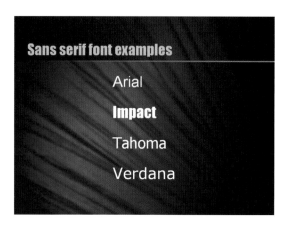

Script fonts

Script fonts are designed to imitate handwriting or calligraphy. They are not italic typefaces and should be used sparingly in presentations. Limit your use of script fonts to large text and headings, as they are generally more difficult to read when projected (Fig. 16.5).

Figure 16.5
Script font examples.

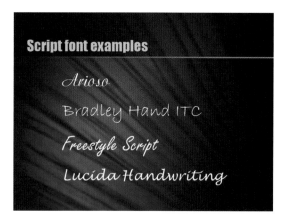

Symbol fonts

Symbol fonts describe a wide range of non-alphabetical fonts and can be used in mathematical formulae or for unique bullet symbols. These fonts come in all different design styles and categories, but most have very limited usage. It might seem clever to use an odd symbol for a bullet point but your audience's focus will be drawn to these symbols and their uniqueness might detract from your message. Keep bullet points simple and straightforward and try to use as few words as possible in each entry (see Chapter 17 for more information about using type in your presentation) (Fig. 16.6).

Figure 16.6
Symbol font examples.

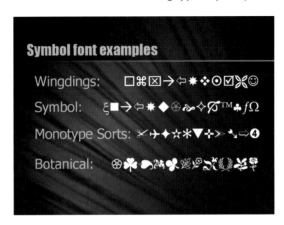

The best use of symbols is for unusual characters that do not appear on a standard keyboard. Thousands of symbols are available, including but certainly not limited to: accented letters, copyright or trademark symbols, monetary symbols, and mathematical symbols.

! ! ! ! ! ! ! ! ! ! ! ! ! ! ! ! Note !

You can customize any toolbar in PowerPoint to include the 'Symbol' shortcut. Select Tools > Customize > Commands and scroll down the list until you see 'Symbol' (Fig. 16.7).

Figure 16.7
Customize commands
dialogue box.

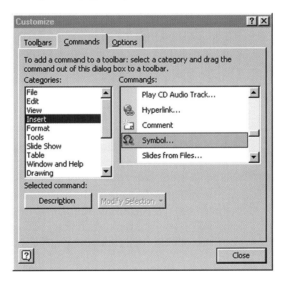

Click and drag this icon to the upper or lower toolbar to lock it in place next to another shortcut. The next time you need a symbol, click the icon and it will open the Symbol dialogue box (Fig. 16.8).

**Decorative or
display fonts**

Decorative or 'display' fonts include everything else that does not neatly fit in the above categories (even though they might or might not have serifs,

Figure 16.8
Symbol dialogue box.

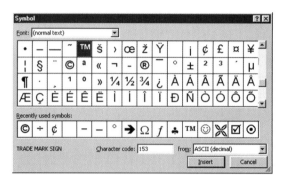

you'll recognize a display font for its distinctive or unique letterforms). These typefaces are full of character and personality and most are too complex to be legible when projected at smaller sizes. Decorative fonts, like serif fonts, should be reserved for headlines, or short statements and phrases (Fig. 16.9).

Figure 16.9
Decorative font examples.

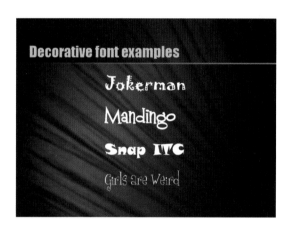

A note about italics

Italic typefaces are slanted to the right, the name coming from the Italian style of writing. A paragraph set in italic type will convey a more relaxed style of prose. Italics help differentiate quotations from other text and they can also be used for soft emphasis of a few words or phrases.

True italic typefaces look more like calligraphy and are designed to complement the rest of the font family. If you have the italic version of a font installed on your system, when you choose the 'italic' format on the toolbar your text should reflect the calligraphic appearance.

! ! ! ! ! ! ! ! ! ! ! ! ! ! ! ! ! ! Note !

In some TrueType families, the text will not automatically convert to the italic version. If you know that you have installed the italic version, simply select it from the font drop down list, and unselect the 'italic' format (Fig. 16.10).

Figure 16.10
Text formatting icons.

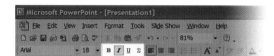

If the font you have chosen does not include a separate version for italics, your text will merely be slanted and you will end up with incorrect sizing and letter spacing. Avoid using computer-generated italics (slanted) and try to use fonts that come with their own unique italic face (Fig. 16.11).

Figure 16.11
Left, corresponding italic type styles; right, incorrect slanted italics.

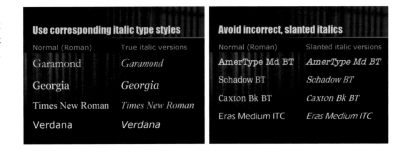

Use corresponding italic type styles		Avoid incorrect, slanted italics	
Normal (Roman)	True italic versions	Normal (Roman)	Slanted italic versions
Garamond	*Garamond*	AmerType Md BT	*AmerType Md BT*
Georgia	*Georgia*	Schadow BT	*Schadow BT*
Times New Roman	*Times New Roman*	Caxton Bk BT	*Caxton Bk BT*
Verdana	*Verdana*	Eras Medium ITC	*Eras Medium ITC*

Capitalization

In pre-computer days, the capital letters used for printing were stored in a separate drawer (or case) from the other letters. The names 'upper case' and 'lower case' derive from this storage system. Text is legible not only because of the individual letters but also because of the flow of letters – we recognize patterns in the spaces between letter combinations (Fig. 16.12).

In this example, the upper word is harder to recognize than the lower one. This is because we recognize the word not just from the letters themselves but also from the flow of the outline of the word.

Capital letters should be used sparingly, for emphasis. You might use all capitals for short titles or headings, but avoid using them for long phrases or bulleted text. Words that appear in all capital letters are not as easy to read as upper and lower case, as the letterform patterns are quite different. Using all capitals can make the text seem to SHOUT OUT LOUD.

Opinions differ as to the appropriate use of capitalization in bulleted lists. Some people capitalize the first word of each bulleted statement whereas others capitalize the first letter of each important word (the worst choice for readability.) Some choose to capitalize each word in titles and headings, and leave everything else lower case. The best advice that we can give is to be consistent throughout your presentation. Choose one rule and stick with it. PowerPoint includes an AutoCorrect tool and you can customize this to suit your preferences. Select Tools > AutoCorrect Options to open the dialogue box.

Figure 16.12 Spaces between letters form patterns.

Text sizing

The main objective with any presentation is communication. Readability and legibility are important keys to communicating. There are no hard rules about the maximum number of words or lines of text you should include on one screen (less is best). When developing your presentation, remember that *all* of your text should be legible to everyone in the audience. If you are putting words on the screen, your audience will naturally want to read them (you should respect that). If you are unsure about readability from the back of the room, project your visuals (in a similar environment whenever possible, including lighting and screen size) and ask a few colleagues to review the text from the back of the room. There are many different settings and types of presentations: a handful of people viewing a laptop, a large classroom or conference room monitor, a small LCD projector to 100 people or less, a large auditorium with rear projection, and so on. Different environments, different lighting, different projectors – each one will impact the appearance of your presentation.

To make your task easier, we can give you a few recommendations about typography for presentations:

- Sans serif fonts are the most legible at any size and Verdana, Tahoma, and Arial are all good choices.
- Titles are usually set larger than 36 points and the main text is generally no smaller than 20 or 24 point (28 point or higher will probably read best).

These are very loose recommendations and sizes will always depend on the distance from your audience. A presentation destined for the web might include much smaller text sizes.

Limit words, increase images

The easiest way to increase the legibility in your presentation is to limit the number of words whenever possible. Pare down your text to include key points only, and not full sentences. Split your slides into two or more when necessary. The visuals should accompany your spoken words and not be a word-for-word repetition of them (your audience will try to read every word on the screen, instead of paying attention to you). We remember images much more readily than bulleted lists and, whenever possible, you should try to convey your ideas graphically (you will find much more on this topic in Chapter 17).

Line spacing

Too little space between bulleted points will make them crowd together and too much space makes the lines seem like separate statements (Fig. 16.13).

Figure 16.13
Tight line spacing makes text difficult to read.

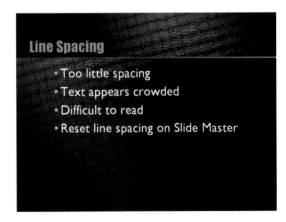

One of the best ways to increase the legibility of text in PowerPoint is to increase the amount of spacing either before or after paragraphs (no need to increase both). Reset the line spacing on the Slide Master, and your changes will take place throughout the presentation (Fig. 16.14).

Figure 16.14
Increased line spacing
improves legibility.

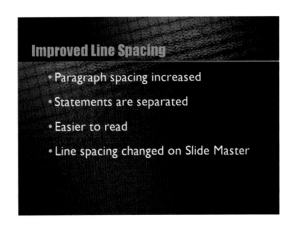

To change the line spacing for your presentation: choose View >
Master > Slide Master, select the text placeholder and then choose
Format > Line Spacing. Increase the spacing 'Before' or 'After paragraph'
to 0.35 lines or higher. Your text might also benefit by decreasing the 'Line
Spacing' to 0.9 or 0.95 lines.

Windows XP Clear Type

To greatly improve the appearance and clarity of your screen font, activate
the Clear Type option in Windows XP. To turn on Clear Type, go to
Control Panel > Display > Appearance > Effects and turn on the
checkbox for 'smooth edges of screen fonts', making sure that the popup
menu reads 'Clear Type'.

Text colors

Your concepts and ideas will be much more legible if they appear at a high
contrast to your background. Dark backgrounds require white or light text
colors and – vice versa – light backgrounds require black or dark text to be
legible. A lighter background (dark text) will work best in a well-lit
environment, whereas a darker background (light text) will project the best
in a room with less light.

It is worth remembering that one in 12 men and one in 200 women are
color blind. The most common problem is red – green color blindness. Avoid
using red and green colors for differentiating or highlighting text. For more
information about color blindness and effective color palettes, see Chapter 17.

Bibliography

Felici J 2003 The complete manual of typography: a guide to setting perfect type.
Adobe Press, Berkeley, CA.
Goodman A 2003 The 7 essentials of graphic design. HOW Design Books, Cincinnati.
Spiekermann E, Ginger EM 2003 Stop stealing sheep and find out how type works,
2nd edn. Adobe Press, Berkeley.
Strizver I 2001 Type rules: the designer's guide to professional typography. North
Light Books, Cincinnati.

Chapter 17

Be different – giving a presentation without PowerPoint®

Terry Irwin and Julie Terberg

Be different

Try presenting without any software! It might seem heresy in a book dedicated to getting the best out of visual presentation software for us to suggest presenting without any software. There is a wonderful PowerPoint® parody of Abraham Lincoln's Gettysburg Address at http://www.norvig.com. Somehow, bullet points just don't convey the same meaning and passion as a well-delivered speech!

So, if you are asked to speak in public, begin by asking yourself, 'Do I need any software at all?' You might want to speak using props instead. This allows you to disconnect yourself from the remote control and get in among your audience. In fact, in medicine the best prop of all is a live patient, and we all teach at the bedside. This works because it keeps the listener interested. You can achieve the same thing in a small group or in a large auditorium. Just choose your prop(s) carefully.

Some speakers like to use handouts instead of showing slides. There is great debate about whether you should hand these out before the talk (then everyone will read them while you are speaking) or at the end. If you hand them out at the end, do you tell the students that you will be doing so (in which case, if they all go to sleep – they can read the handout) or tell them as you hand them out at the end (in which case they all take their own notes as they go along and do not hear all that you say). Hmm, as we say this is controversial!

Some teachers give the handout to the students well in advance and let them read up the material for the talk. Others will hand out a template with questions for the students to try to answer in advance, to provide a basis for discussion.

A recent innovation is to tell the students what the problem is, direct them to resources to solve it and let them run the session themselves. This is the ultimate in problem-based learning but requires considerable planning and skill to make it work.

You have to decide which system works best for you and your audience. Trial and error is still one of the best ways to learn.

For most occasions, visual props on a projector remain the best way of imparting information. Whereas PowerPoint remains the ultimate tool for creating slideshows, there are occasions when you will want to try something different. This might be because you want to put the slideshow online and you are not sure whether all your viewers will have PowerPoint viewer, or just because you want to be different. You might want something that will run itself or that has text effects that cannot be created in PowerPoint. Vive la difference!

Creating a PDF slideshow using Photoshop Elements®

The advantage of the PDF (portable document format) is that the graphics render well and can be resized to any size; also, a free reader is available to enable anyone with a computer (PC, Mac, Linux, PDA, Palm) to view the files.

It is not as easy to add text using this technique, so it is best reserved for occasions when you want to put together a series of images. This might be for a question-and-answer session with students, or in an examination.

To begin, we need to assemble all of the images in one folder; in this case we have done this for you in the folder 'pdf' located in the Chapter 17 folder of the CD. If you are doing this yourself, put all your images in one folder.

Select File > Batch Processing and the dialogue box shown in Figure 17.1 will open.

Figure 17.1
Batch Processing dialogue box.

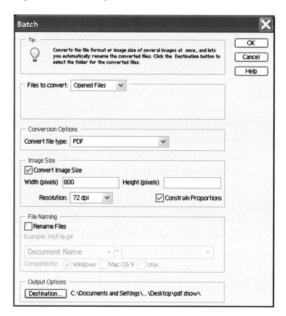

Set the choices as illustrated. Click on 'Destination' and then choose your desktop. Now click on 'Create new folder' and call the folder 'pdf show', and hit 'OK'.

Relax; all that flashing is Photoshop Elements resizing the images to be 800 pixels across. Now close the file browser and any open image files.

If you want to add a text slide, just open a new file in Photoshop Elements and set the size to 800 × 600 pixels. Add the text using the Text tool and then save the image (as a .pdf) in the same folder as your other slides.

Select File > Automation Tools > PDF Slideshow. Click 'Browse' and then navigate to the folder containing your images and select them all

(Ctrl A). Under output file click 'Choose', give your file a name and select a location to save it. You can reorder files in the 'Source files' list by dragging them up or down as desired. If you want the show to loop continuously, select 'loop after last page'. Choose from one of the available transitions and then click 'OK'.

Now open the file that you have created with the Adobe® Acrobat Reader®. If you do not already have it installed, you can download the free program at http://www.adobe.com/products/acrobat/readstep2.html.

Alternative presentation software programs

Believe it or not, there are a lot of people who do *not* use PowerPoint to create their presentations. There are many alternative programs to choose from. You might have heard of Lotus® Freelance Graphics®, Corel Presentations®, Harvard Graphics®, or Star Office®, just to name a few. If you work on a Mac, you might currently be working with Apple Keynote®.

Perhaps your company, department, or hospital already has other presentation software in place and you are required to learn this program to produce your images. Or you might already be familiar with a professional quality animation program, like Flash®, and prefer to work with the tools you know.

Relax, you are not alone, and you can produce beautiful and effective presentations. As you read through this book you will notice that much of the text is devoted to preparing content and images for your presentation. And some of the tools in PowerPoint will be very similar to those in alternative programs – you might even find that basic keyboard shortcuts are the same. Certain presentation programs, such as Star Office, will even import and export .ppt files, so any PowerPoint files from the CD will be compatible.

PowerPoint is basically a presentation assembly and delivery tool and it cannot make you a better presenter. Use your new knowledge from this book to develop a presentation with whatever program you happen to have available!

Chapter 18

Effective presentations – from concept to delivery

Julie Terberg and Terry Irwin

'An honest tale speeds best being plainly told' (William Shakespeare, *Richard III*)

A great speaker can captivate an audience with voice and body language alone, the rest of us need good supporting material to assist us in communicating our ideas.

Most presentations are designed to achieve one of two functions: to inform or to persuade. No matter what your subject is, the key to an effective presentation is 'communication'. You are trying to communicate information to an audience. That information may be in the form of research results, training or educational materials, reports, or why they should purchase a product or service. Whatever material you are presenting, you should strive to communicate that information clearly.

Planning

An effective presentation begins with the planning stage. Plan for all aspects of your presentation by asking yourself the following questions early:

- 'What is my topic?'
- 'Who is my audience?'
- 'What do I want the audience to learn from me?'
- 'What is the purpose of this presentation?'
- 'How will I deliver the presentation?'
- 'How much time do I have to present?'

Topic and purpose

Using the answers to these questions, you can create a plan for your presentation. Define your topic by writing it down. What is the basic theme of your presentation? Next, define your audience.

Every aspect of your presentation will be affected by your audience. Your preparation for a formal research presentation to a large international

161

medical meeting in a 2000-seat auditorium will be very different from that for a talk to potential doctors and dentists at your old high school.

What is the audience's current knowledge of your subject? Will the information be of relevance to them in their everyday lives or are you informing them for some other reason? For example, a talk on 'recent advances in our understanding of why misfolded prion protein in the cytosol is toxic and causes neurodegenerative disease' given at a neurological research meeting will assume a very different level of knowledge compared with a similar talk given to a local neurology patient charity fundraising group!

What will the audience want to learn about your topic? What information do you want to communicate to this audience? Are you trying to inform them, amuse them, or persuade them? Keep your answers in mind when you are developing your visuals.

Environment

Are you presenting to a large group in an auditorium or to a few people around a conference table? The size of the screen, the size of your audience, and their distance from the screen should be determined before you begin developing the visuals. As a general rule, the larger the set, the more formal you need to make your style. You will find it hard to interact with more than 30 or 40 people, unless you are a skilled speaker.

Respect your audience and make sure that your typography and graphics are large enough for everyone to read. Along with the venue and the audience, you need to consider the room lighting. Will the room be well lit or have low-level lighting?

Time limit

When planning your presentation, determine how much time you will have to communicate your point. As you develop the content, you will want to practice how long it takes to go through each slide, pacing yourself in a slightly heightened conversational tone. Whenever appropriate, plan enough time to answer questions from the audience.

Preparation

Gather materials

Before you begin designing or developing your presentation, gather all the existing materials required to support your subject matter. This might include logos, charts, graphs, statistics, quotations, photographs, existing slides, or any other visuals that will help you communicate. Appropriately chosen images and well-developed graphics will help you convey your message much more effectively than bullet point after bullet point of text.

Which version of PowerPoint®?

We will assume that you will be presenting using PowerPoint, although there are other options. Which version is available on the machine from which you will project the presentation? If you do not know, either find out or assume it is no more than Office 2000®. This is because some of the effects that you might choose to use in PowerPoint from Office XP® or even PowerPoint 2003 will not be supported.

Typically, older versions of PowerPoint do not support transparency (Fig. 18.1).

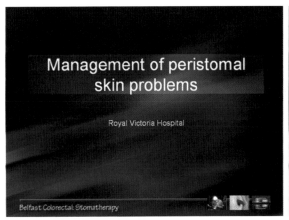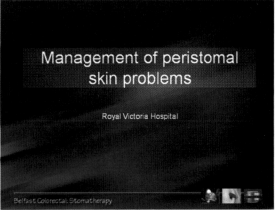

Figure 18.1   Left, a PowerPoint 2002 slide using transparency behind the title; right, the same slide shown in PowerPoint 2000. Note that the transparency has been replaced by a stippled box, which makes the text difficult to read.

Making an initial impact

Those first few slides are crucial. You need to grab the attention of your audience.

Humor can make or break a presentation. Good speakers can carry it off but they are a minority. An occasional caricature or cartoon can also be useful but never overdo this.

Make sure that your humor works! If you are planning to use a joke, first test it on friends and family or on a practice audience.

If humor is not your strong point, try an opening with impact. A colleague began a memorable ATLS talk on trauma some years ago with an image of a motor vehicle accident in which a young girl died. He asked the audience what injuries she might have died from. When he pointed out that her only problem was an obstructed airway, he grabbed the audience's attention right away.

You might begin by quoting an expert on the subject who is known to the audience. The more relevant, novel, fascinating, or controversial your opening quotation is, the greater its impact. Be outrageous, it certainly grabs their attention! Be aware, however, that outrageous must still be politically correct and definitely not offensive.

Develop an outline

The next step in preparation should be to develop an outline, listing the points you want to cover and the order in which you will present them. This is the presentation structure. You can think of it as a skeleton that you will build upon. The outline can be very rough at this stage. As you expand these ideas into slides and rehearse your timing, you might find items that need to be cut, added, or revised. Keep focused as you develop the outline and remember your main objective for the presentation.

Now for the set-up; tell them what you are going to tell them! (Once you have finished your presentation, you will want to summarize this again.)

Write a script

It can be beneficial to develop a script from your outline. For certain high-level presentations, a writer will carefully craft each word of a script and the presenter will read them from a teleprompter. During these high-level presentations, an audiovisual team handles the presentation graphics and video, advancing them at predetermined points on the script. Although this might be overkill for your situation, writing a script *can* help you determine which words you will use in front of the audience, better preparing you for an effective delivery.

Your script can be as simple as a list of certain points you want to cover for each visual, or as complete as a word-for-word document that you will rehearse and memorize. Either way, practicing with some sort of script will make your final presentation delivery much smoother and easier.

When you present, it is better to work from an outline on cue cards than from a full script. This makes the flow of your narrative more natural and conversational. It allows a little flexibility; say if the audience reacts to a comment. Most importantly, it avoids the embarrassment of losing your place!

Storyboard

Whether you work from an outline or a full script, developing a storyboard can be a key step in preparing an effective presentation. A storyboard is a graphic depiction or description of a frame or series of frames arranged in sequence.

These frames, or slides, can be sketched out on paper, with notes about which supporting images you will use, how you might arrange the elements, what images you still need to acquire, and so on.

! ! ! ! ! ! ! ! ! ! ! ! ! ! ! ! ! *Tip !*

Use PowerPoint handouts for your blank storyboard. Create three blank slides and select handouts for printing, three to a page, this will give you blank rules on which to make any storyboard notes (Fig. 18.2).

We are not suggesting that you always need to develop a script or a storyboard; an outline might be enough for you to get started. However, if you are new to presentation process, or are looking for ways to improve your skills, a storyboard can be a great tool for organizing your thoughts and ideas before you begin development.

Closing

'Make sure you have finished speaking before your audience has finished listening.' (Dorothy Sarnoff)

You need to plan the end of your presentation just as meticulously as the beginning. Make sure that you reach this point in the correct time. Nothing is worse than a speaker who runs over – except a speaker who runs over so badly they are stopped by the person chairing the meeting. The whole impact of your presentation is lost at that point and people only remember that you were the guy who liked the sound of his own voice!

Tell your audience that you are about to finish. Summarize your main points briefly (don't give the whole talk again). Leave the audience with a message.

If you are presenting research data, make sure that this message is supported by your data. All too often a talk is spoiled at the final slide by a statement that is wishful and cannot be supported by the data presented. This often

Figure 18.2
Create a few blank slides in PowerPoint and then print handouts, three to a page. Use these blank storyboard pages to develop the contents for your slides.

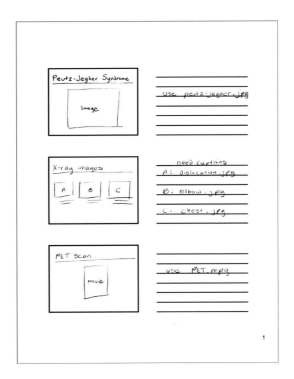

entails dramatic claims that the therapy or technique presented (in 20 laboratory mice) is the treatment of choice for some complex condition.

Development

Template selection

Now you're ready to begin working in PowerPoint (or another presentation development program). You will need to determine which template you will use. Perhaps it will be a template that you have been provided with, or one that you have designed yourself. You should know from reading Chapter 6 that standard templates just won't do. It doesn't take much time to develop a unique, attractive, and appropriate template.

When choosing or designing a template, consider your final presentation venue. If you will be projecting your visuals in a dark room, use a medium to dark background with white or light-colored text. Conversely, if you are presenting in a well-lit room, use a lighter background with black or dark-colored text.

!!!!!!!!!!!!!!!!!! Note ! Refer to Chapters 6 and 16 for more information.

Always remember that the template is just that. It does not convey the message of your presentation, just gives it a professional look. You must balance the time you take in preparing the template against the time taken to put together the content. It might be better to take time out to develop some templates when a talk is not due and use one of these as needed. It is always tempting to spend hours making a presentation look really good and not enough time on the message.

However, a bad template can be very distracting. As a general rule, the templates that come with PowerPoint can be divided into two groups: those that look good but are used by everyone (typically 'Blue Diagonal' or 'Stream') and those that are just downright ghastly! We rarely use them. If you are giving a simple talk to a few immediate colleagues, you could simply choose to use a plain background. Wasting time on a template in such situations is pure self-indulgence!

Never, ever, use the templates with special effects such as animated lights. They look good when you see them for the first time but they distract an audience and, by the tenth slide, will start to irritate them!

Simplifying your slide content

The best one-word advice you'll ever receive regarding presentation development is 'simplify'. With communication as your key presentation objective, everything that you put up on the screen should be legible and visible to everyone in your audience. When you simplify your visuals to include just the key points, you help your audience to understand your message. It is a common mistake to put everything that you want to say about a topic on one visual. This produces cluttered, disorganized slides, and smaller, hard-to-read text.

Start by splitting-up complex slides. You do not need to squeeze all of your ideas about one subject onto one slide. We have all seen slides full of 12 point text combined with multiple charts and photographs, a three-line title, subtitle, and illegible footnotes (Fig. 18.3).

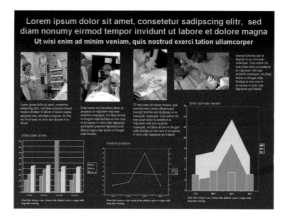

Figure 18.3
Do not follow this example. Too much information clutters the slide and makes it more difficult for your audience to read (photography by Royal College of Surgeons Photographic Studios).

Your audience will try to read every word on the screen. Keep it simple and they will listen to you instead.

Legibility is a key to communication. By limiting the number of words on a slide, you automatically make it easier to read (larger typography). Use simple statements and phrases on your slides, not full sentences. You should not be reading the slides word for word. Why would the audience want or need to listen to you when they could simply read the screen? Presentation slides should be a summary of your key points, with images, graphics, charts, and so on that support and reinforce those key points. Your spoken words should be the focus of the presentation, not the visuals. Simplify your charts

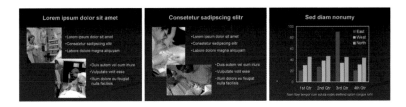

Figure 18.4
Split up complex visuals into multiple slides, try and keep one or two ideas per slide. Simplify chart information by reducing the number of labels, losing the three-dimensional bars and outlines, and enlarging all text (photography by Royal College of Surgeons Photographic Studios).

and graphs whenever possible by reducing the number of points on the scale and the amount of text on the chart (Fig. 18.4).

When simplifying your slides, try to break-up information into smaller-sized bits. Can you present the material graphically instead of using bullet points? We are a visual society and, as such, we remember visual information much better than written words. Exercise your imagination and develop your left-brain thinking, sharpen your pencil and start sketching – it can be as simple as a couple of boxes and could progress to a much more sophisticated illustration (if you are so inclined). The point here is to avoid too many words – use images to make your point whenever possible (Fig. 18.5).

Figure 18.5
The slide on the left is very wordy and not very appealing. Adding images and breaking up the information into columns makes it more appealing and easier to read and comprehend (right). Note that the bulleted text has also been edited.

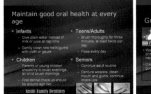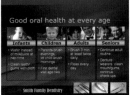

! ! ! ! ! ! ! ! ! ! ! ! ! ! ! ! Note !

When compiling your supporting images and graphics, avoid selecting clip art, which tends to look 'cute' and amateurish. Stick with photographic images and objects. There are many good resources for professional quality images (see Chapter 9). Whatever images you decide to use, make sure you optimize them for use in PowerPoint.

! ! ! ! ! ! ! ! ! ! ! ! ! ! ! ! Note !

See Chapter 4 for information on resizing your images, and Chapter 14 for tips on improving or altering your images.

PowerPoint comes with a large selection of office clip art. It is a matter of personal taste, but we generally avoid it. If you choose to use clip art, use it sparingly and try not to mix illustration styles.

Slide layout and design

Your presentation template is not called a 'template' for nothing. It has been formatted with typography choices, color schemes, bullet point choices, line spacing, and a layout scheme (justification and position). You should try to follow this formatting throughout your presentation. Keep your title position and size consistent. Use the bullet points and spacing set up on the slide master. Select colors from the template color scheme. Apply the same outline and drop shadow treatment to similar objects. If you develop a graphic treatment for a repeating element, such as headings, tables, or charts, apply this new style consistently.

!!!!!!!!!!!!!!!!!!!!!*Tip!*   Get to know the 'Pick Up and Apply' tools in PowerPoint (see Chapter 7).

After you start developing your presentation, you may find that you need to change font sizes. Make these corrections to the Slide Master so that all the slides are consistent throughout the presentation. Do not change font sizes slide by slide. However, as we keep repeating, if there is so much text that it will not fit easily, you probably need less text, not a smaller (less legible) font.

Along with consistent elements and placement, you should use your guidelines to create a ½-inch (approximately) margin around the perimeter of your Slide Master. Keep the guidelines visible as you are developing your slides, and use them to remind you not to put any important information too close to the edge of the screen. Type 'Ctrl G' to open the Grid and Guides dialogue box, and hold the 'Ctrl' key and drag any guideline to make a copy (Fig. 18.6).

Figure 18.6
Use guidelines in PowerPoint to establish outer margins and other key alignment positions.

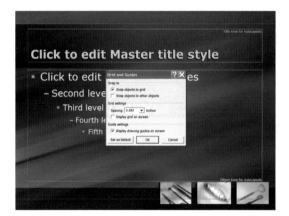

Take the time to align your graphics and text. PowerPoint includes a great drawing tool called 'Align and Distribute'. With your graphics selected, choose Draw > Align and Distribute. You can even peel this toolbar off of the 'Draw' menu and leave it on your desktop for quicker access. Select the objects you wish to align and choose your alignment options from the toolbar. The distribution tools on this menu will create even spacing between all of the selected objects.

Consistency and proofreading

Whichever capitalization rules you decide to use (first letter of each line, every important word, etc.) follow these rules on every slide. If you are using abbreviations, make sure your audience will know their full meaning. Always finish your presentation with complete spell checking and proofreading, you might even want to pass a hard copy along to a colleague for another pair of eyes to read through. You can be sure that your audience will notice any spelling mistakes and typos on your slides.

Color blindness (color deficiencies)

To have a truly effective presentation you must consider everyone in your audience. To this end, it is helpful to remember that one in 12 men and one in 200 women are color blind. The most common problem is red–green color blindness. Consider the most common color blindness traits when developing your slides. Avoid using red and green together and avoid combinations of yellow, browns, and greens (Fig. 18.7).

Figure 18.7
High contrast produces the most legible presentation text. Follow these simple guidelines when developing your template color palette.

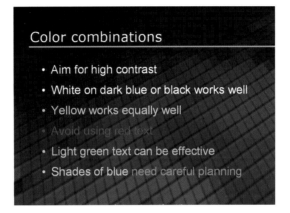

In general, we have tried to avoid too many web links in this book, because they are so often broken when you go looking for them. However, if you want to know more about color blindness, there is a very informative site at http://www.webexhibits.org/causesofcolor.

Slide transitions and animation

Slide transitions look better when they are simple and clean. PowerPoint includes some really distracting transitions, such as the 'strips' 'checkerboard', and 'blinds'. Just because they are included doesn't mean you should use them. If you have an older version of PowerPoint, try to stick with the 'wipe' transitions, the 'box in, box out', and the 'split' transitions. Choose a transition type for each different type of layout in your presentation, and repeat them, changing the direction of the transition for more effect. If you are using PowerPoint 2002, try the 'fade smoothly' transition – it is a clean and simple fade from one slide to the next. If you are used to selecting 'random' transitions, stop. It is better to select all of your slides and apply one simple transition, such as a 'wipe right' or 'fade smoothly', than to use the mishmash you get using 'random' effects. The easiest way to program slide transitions is by using the Slide Sorter view. Select View > Slide Sorter or choose the icon on the lower left of your screen. If you are short on time, you can type 'Ctrl A' to select all of the slides and apply one type of transition for all (Fig. 18.8).

Keep transitions simple and repeat a few types throughout your presentation. Do not animate everything on every slide – this is distracting and unprofessional. It is better to choose a few key elements to animate or build onto your slides. Animated builds can be very effective but there should be a reason or purpose for building the elements, not just for entertainment! The same advice applies to sound effects; avoid using them unless you feel they are an important part of your message.

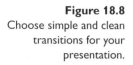

Figure 18.8
Choose simple and clean transitions for your presentation.

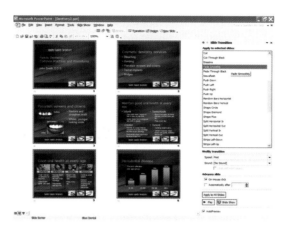

Delivery

Rehearse

Rehearse, rehearse, and rehearse again. You should be comfortable presenting all of your visuals, and familiar with the information on each slide. It can be very helpful to practice using a printed version of each of your visuals. Use the 'Notes Pages' in PowerPoint to type in your script or key points for discussion, and then print these notes pages to refer to during your delivery.

As you practice, check your timing. Can you present everything within the allotted time for your final presentation? Are you falling short and need to expand certain areas or do you keep running out of time and need to cut something? Remember to speak naturally, pausing before and after key points.

Use cue cards

Never read from a full-text script. This will make your delivery dry and monotonous. The spontaneity and the flaws of natural speech will keep your subject alive and your audience awake. We prefer to use cue cards or no prompts at all.

Make it flow

Your presentation will probably consist of several sections. You will need to find ways to link these. The transitions between these elements can be filled with simple sentences: 'Now that you have a clear understanding of the etiology of…, let's move on to how we treat it'. Or you can summarize your content to date: 'So we've discussed these five causes of… and you have learned that… is the most common, now let's look at treatment options'. If you are a beginner, plan these transitions.

Questions

Whenever appropriate, leave sufficient time for questions and answers from the audience. Plan for possible questions about the material you are presenting, you might even want to have a list of potential questions and answers prepared ahead of time.

When someone asks a question, it is not always possible for everyone to hear it. Get into the habit of repeating the question loudly enough for the entire audience to hear before starting your response.

Always treat questioners with respect, even if they don't deserve it! Thank them for their question and answer it fully. Wait for the full question to be given and never interrupt. If you find it hard to answer questions because you are nervous, write the question down as it is asked.

Tone, volume, and speed

Try to give your talk in a relaxed conversational tone. It should be loud enough to be heard but not so loud as to be irritating. The cardinal sin is to speak too quietly to be heard.

You can vary the loudness of your voice for effect. Speak slowly and quietly to get attention. This can be a good way to get the audience to pay attention at the start. Alternatively, you might start loud, with a list of facts that hook the audience because of their impact factor.

You can also vary the tempo to add emphasis. Speak quickly to add excitement or slowly to draw the audience in, such as with a sad story. Use pauses to allow important points to sink in.

Body language

Your body language is also important. Don't stand behind a lectern if you can avoid it. Indeed, if you are very anxious, you might make the lectern shake and the rattling of the microphone will distract the audience!

Feel free to walk about if you can, making plenty of eye contact with the audience. This makes you feel and look confident. Remember to make eye contact with as much of the room as possible, the back as well as the front. If you are nervous about this, look at their foreheads rather than their eyes; to the audience the difference is imperceptible.

Gestures can be useful but don't wave your hands about too much. Stand up straight and look like you mean it!

Get in among them! If you can, especially in a small room, walk in among the audience and interact with them if the subject matter allows this.

Avoid irritating the audience. There are many ways of doing this:

- Repeated words or phrases ('OK', 'um').
- Swaying, rocking, or clinging to the lectern for grim death.
- Pacing like a caged bear.
- Hands in pockets (although occasionally this can be effective).
- Making funny noises (lip smacking, throat clearing, sighing).
- Apologizing: never apologize unless everything has gone *completely* pear-shaped! Certainly never apologize for being nervous.
- Fidgeting, playing with jewelry, face rubbing, stroking your hair.

Tips for running your presentation

When developing your presentation slides you will want to consider how to begin and end your presentation. If you are the only presenter at the event, do you want to have an introductory slide up on the screen as the audience enters the room? Or would you prefer a presentation title, or a logo perhaps? Consider the closing slide as well. You might want to include a slide that says 'Questions and answers' or 'Q&A'. A summary slide might be enough to close your presentation, or you could chose to add a simple 'thank you' up on the screen as you thank your audience before they leave the presentation.

When delivering your PowerPoint presentation, you have a few choices for navigating between slides.

- Go to the next slide:
  - click the mouse
  - type 'N'
  - press 'Spacebar' or 'Enter'
  - use the right or down arrow
  - right-click, and on the shortcut menu, click 'Next'.
- Go to the previous slide:
  - press 'Backspace'
  - type 'P'
  - use the left or up arrow
  - right-click, and on the shortcut menu, click 'Previous'.
- Go to a specific slide:
  - type the slide number, and then press 'Enter'
  - right-click, point to 'Go' on the shortcut menu, then point to 'By Title,' and click the slide you want.
- See previously viewed slide:
  - right-click, point to 'Go' on the shortcut menu, and then click 'Previously Viewed'.

For more information about running your presentation, see the 'Microsoft® PowerPoint Help' section under the 'Help' menu in PowerPoint.

Presentation day

Dress

How do you dress? First impressions are vital. A useful guide is to dress just a little more formally than the audience. So for a presentation at a job interview, it has got to be a suit and tie; for women a smart business suit.

On the other hand, at a workshop with an audience composed of trainees, where there will be a relaxed style, a casual open-necked shirt is best.

Just occasionally it works the other way round. A psychologist at a meeting of power-dressing, high-earning, plastic surgeons might convey just the image they are seeking by dressing down – a crumpled linen suit and tee shirt. This takes careful judgment!

Jewelry

Jewelry should be kept to a minimum. Discreet earrings, brooches, and necklaces are fine. Large dangling earrings can be very distracting. Women should avoid bracelets, particularly those enormous, noisy metal ones that speakers are so fond of fiddling with as they speak. They make an audience want to scream!

At the venue

So you arrive at the venue, CD in hand. You should check-in with the projectionist or IT support team and run through your presentation as soon as possible to make sure that it works. If you have left the video on your desktop on the other side of the Atlantic there just might be time to get it sent by e-mail!

Make sure that the CD or disk is clearly labeled and that the support team understands when and where you are presenting.

Now go to the podium and make sure that you know how all of the controls work. How do you advance a slide and how do you go back? Can you control the sound, light and heat – how? Can the projectionist hear you?

Is there a laser pointer, does it work? Good presenters carry their own laser pointer; never lend it to the speaker before you because they will keep their finger on the button and run the battery down just before you speak!

If you are going to use a laser pointer, use it only to make a point. Do not wave it over your slide and never point it at the audience – unless you know exactly where the chap with diabetic retinopathy is sitting and you have a very steady hand!

Figure 18.9
Never point the laser pointer at the audience.

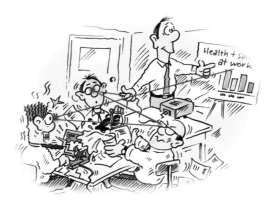

Of course, not all talks are given in large auditoria with IT support. More often you will do all the work yourself. Here the approach is different because you are in control.

First, notice how the seats are arranged and if it is possible for you to rearrange them. You might want an informal semicircle for group discussion, or a more formal row arrangement for a heads-up lecture. Sort out the light, heat, and sound before the audience arrives. Get the laptop and projector up and running and make sure you know how to control both. Ensure that the screensaver on the laptop is off! Navigate to your first slide and then relax. Have a coffee!

Waiting for the audience to settle in their seats can be awkward. Use the time to interact with them and get them warmed up. Chat about the course, their prior experience of the subject, and their expectations of your talk. Try to learn a few names. This can help to personalize your presentation.

'Good morning, I'm John Milligan. I'm a clinical chemist here at the University Hospital and I'm going to discuss acid–base balance with you today. Mary was telling me that you found the lectures last semester on acid–base balance daunting! So I'm going to keep this very simple and practical and by coffee time, you will all be experts!'

With this one opening sentence you are achieving several goals. You make your subject relevant to this audience and you explain what they are going to learn. You add a tiny bit of humor – in the correct environment the suggestion that you will turn a group of students into experts in an hour will usually get a response that breaks the ice.

There are a few tricks that are not in any PowerPoint manuals, which are very useful in this sort of informal setting. When you pause your talk to discuss a point you can show a blank slide. To show a pure white slide, type 'W' and to show a black slide type 'B'. Just retype the letter or hit 'Enter' to return to the slide show.

It is also helpful to have a complete list of all of your slides, and perhaps extra slides showing answers to questions you might anticipate. If you need to show a particular slide you can then go straight to it by typing the slide number and return.

Follow up

If you choose to leave handouts for your audience, take the time to make sure all of the slides are legible on the hard copies. PowerPoint 2002 includes a 'Print Preview' feature: select File > Print Preview. This allows you to see how your slides will look when printed in grayscale, with the background dropped out (Fig. 18.10). If you decide to pare down your presentation, or change any of the colors or graphics to improve your handouts, remember to 'Save as' a copy and don't save over your original version.

Figure 18.10
PowerPoint 2002 Print Preview feature allows you to see on screen how your presentation will look when printed.

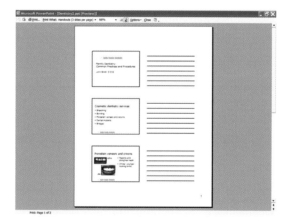

We recommend distributing handouts after your presentation because they become a distraction to your audience and take the focus away from your delivery. Some audience members will look ahead through the handouts, instead of listening to you. However, there are always those instances when handouts are deemed essential and might even assist a presenter in communicating a particular message.

In some circumstances you might want to give the handout to the audience well in advance of your presentation. This works well with an interactive tutorial.

Archiving and evaluation

Save your presentation, especially if you have made last-minute changes, and keep an archival copy on your preferred method of storage (external hard drive, CD, disk, etc.).

If you want to improve for your next presentation, take the time to evaluate yourself. Did your audience understand you and could they clearly read all of your visuals? Did your slides help you communicate your information effectively? Were you well-rehearsed and comfortable during delivery? Were you prepared for all of the questions received after your presentation? If you had another opportunity to present the same material, what would you change? Keeping notes on all of these questions will better prepare you for your next presentation.

Chapter 19

Cool tips and techniques

Julie Terberg and Terry Irwin

If you have read all of the chapters preceding this one, you will have learned basic techniques for manipulating, optimizing, and saving your digital images, as well as techniques for creating an effective presentation. In this chapter we're going to go beyond the basics and show you some interesting and eye-catching tricks that you can apply in your presentations to make them stand out from the rest.

Some of the effects are accomplished using Photoshop Elements®, the rest are produced with PowerPoint® 2002.

Tricks with Photoshop Elements

Image-filled text

You might want to fill a headline or bold statement with a great digital image. In the following example, the image of a spine is perfect for a vertically stacked headline of the word 'SPINE'. This is a fairly simple effect to achieve in Photoshop Elements.

Open the file 'SpineImage.jpg' from the Chapter 19 folder on the CD.

Select the Vertical Type tool from the fly-out Text menu on the Photoshop Elements Toolbox (click and hold the 'T' icon) (Fig. 19.1). The foreground color does not matter for this exercise. Select the Top Align Text icon from the Options bar (Fig. 19.2). Place the cursor just below the top of the 'SpineImage' box. Type the word 'SPINE' in all capital letters. It is best to use a large, bold, serif font; we used Arial Black at a point size of '95'. In fact, you can drag the box surrounding the text to make it fill the canvas. If necessary, use the Move tool ('V') to center the text within the image. Save your file, giving it a new name such as 'SpineText.psd'.

In the Layers palette, click and drag the Background layer to the small folder icon in the lower right (create a new layer) or select Layer > New > Layer via Copy. Still in the Layers palette, click and drag this new 'Background copy' layer and move it above the 'SPINE' layer. Next, make the Background layer invisible by clicking the 'eye' icon to the left of the layer name. With the Background copy layer selected (not the text, this is important), type 'Ctrl G' or select Layer > Group with Previous. The word 'SPINE' should now be filled with the image.

You could leave the word as is and save your file for your presentation or poster design. For this example, we will add a few more enhancements.

Figure 19.1
Vertical Type tool.

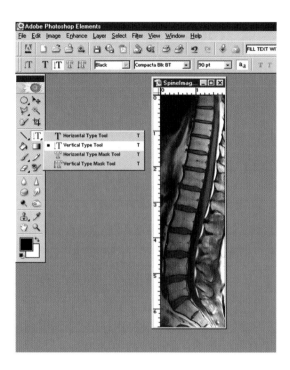

Figure 19.2
Top Align Text tool.

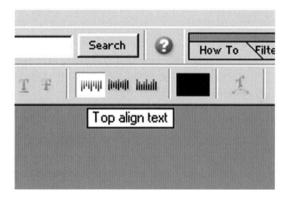

Double-click on the Background layer in the Layers palette and give it a new name, such as 'lighter spine image'. Edit the hue/saturation for this layer by typing 'Ctrl U' (Enhance > Adjust Color > Hue/Saturation). Slide the Lightness slider to approximately '+60' (Fig. 19.3).

The finishing touch for our 'SPINE' headline is a text layer drop shadow. Select the SPINE layer from the Layers palette and then the Layer Styles palette (Window > Layer Styles). Choose 'Drop Shadow' from the popup menu and click any of the drop shadow styles to apply it to your text. For the example, we have chosen 'low' (Fig. 19.4). If you choose any of the other drop shadow styles and change your mind, you can clear the effect by clicking on the Clear Style icon in the upper right corner of the Layer Styles window.

Figure 19.3
Hue/saturation dialogue box.

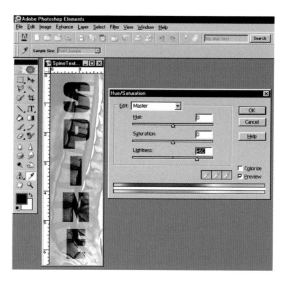

Figure 19.4
Spine Text final image.

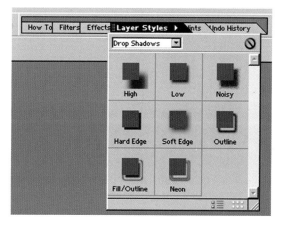

Layer styles

Photoshop Elements has many preprogrammed 'layer styles' that you can apply to enhance typography and graphic elements. Open the file 'finepoint.tif' from the chapter folder on the CD.

Type 'T' to select the Text tool, click the cursor near the top of the image and type the word 'precision'. Choose whichever font you want for this exercise; we selected 30-point Arial Black. On the Text Options bar, set the 'text color' to white. Click the cursor near the top of the image and type the word 'precision'. With the Text layer selected in the Layers palette, open the Layer Styles window and choose 'Bevels' from the pop-up menu.

Click on each of the bevel styles to sample the effect on the word 'precision'. Select the 'simple pillow' bevel and save your work with a new name such as 'precision.psd'.

You can edit the Layer Effects that you apply to your images to customize their final appearance. Double-click on the italicized 'f' in the Text layer to bring up the Style Settings dialogue box (or select Layer > Layer Style > Style Settings). For this particular bevel effect, you can change the lighting angle, the bevel direction, and the bevel size.

In the Layer Effects window, select 'Outer Glows' from the pop-up menu. Click on the 'Noisy' effect to apply it to the word 'precision'. Double-click on the italicized 'f' in the Text Layer, and slide the Outer Glow Size to '40 px' (Fig. 19.5).

Figure 19.5
Outer Glow Style settings (photography by Royal College of Surgeons Photographic Studios).

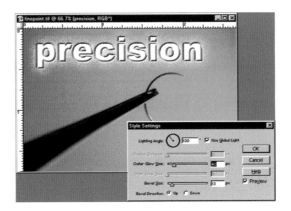

The last step in this exercise is to change the 'Blending mode' for the Text layer. You change the layer-blending mode to affect how the pixel colors blend with the layers beneath. In the Layers palette, with the Text layer selected, click the small black arrow next to the word 'normal' (Fig. 19.6). Choose 'multiply' and notice how the white text becomes transparent to the background image. Type 'V' or select the Move tool and move the word 'precision' to the center of the image. Save your work (Fig. 19.7).

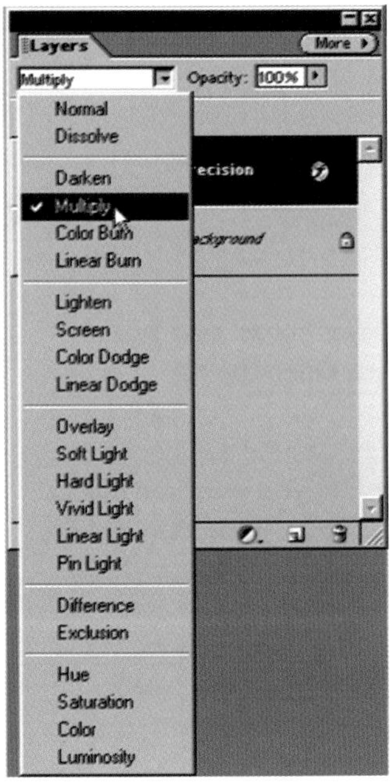

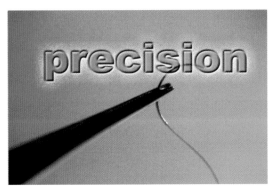

Figure 19.6   Layer blending mode.

Figure 19.7   Final 'precision' text and image (photography by Royal College of Surgeons Photographic Studios).

Using filters

There are so many filters included with Photoshop Elements that the best way to learn how they will affect your images is to do a lot of experimenting. Try out some of the filters on your own images and compare results.

Open the file 'RCScrop.tif' from the chapter folder on the CD. Double-click on the Background layer and select 'OK' to make this an editable layer. Open the Filters tab, Windows > Filters and choose 'Artistic' from the pop-up menu. Scroll down to the bottom of this list of filters, choose 'Watercolor' and click the 'Apply' button in the top right corner. The Watercolor dialogue box will appear. Slide the Brush Detail to '14', the Shadow Intensity to '0', and then click 'OK' (Fig. 19.8).

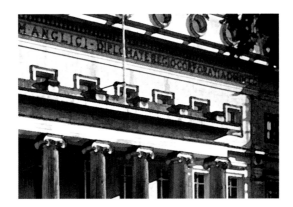

Figure 19.8
Close-up of watercolor filter applied to image (photography by Royal College of Surgeons Photographic Studios).

Feathered edge photo

You can combine filters, effects, and layer styles to create custom images from one original photo. You might want to apply an artistic filter and add an interesting frame from the Effects menu. Try it for yourself: open the file 'surgery.tif' from the chapter folder. Open the 'Filters' window, select 'Artistic' from the pop-up menu, and then Apply 'Smudge Stick'. On the Smudge Stick options menu, change the Stroke Length to '10', the Highlight Area to '10', and the Intensity to '2'. Click 'OK' to accept. Next, open the Effects window and select 'Frames' from the pop-up menu. Apply the 'Strokes' frame from the list and watch the program do the work (Fig. 19.9).

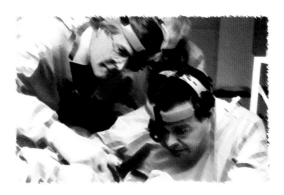

Figure 19.9
Smudge Stick filter and Strokes Frame effect (photography by Royal College of Surgeons Photographic Studios).

It is wise not to mix too many image styles in a presentation. If you decide to use a filter or effect on your images, keep its use consistent throughout your visuals. The example shows four different images with the Film Grain filter and Teal Photographic Effect applied to each (Fig. 19.10). These images could be used as accents within a presentation.

Figure 19.10
Film Grain filter and Teal Photographic Layer style (photography by Royal College of Surgeons Photographic Studios).

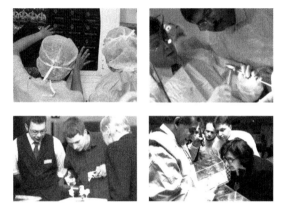

Most of the effects applied in Photoshop Elements will distort the clarity of your original and are intended mainly as a design treatment. If clarity is important for your images, steer clear of any of the image or photographic effects.

Tricks with PowerPoint 2002

Fill effects and transparency

PowerPoint 2002 includes a host of new features. One of the nicest additions to the program is the ability to fill objects and shapes with truly transparent colors, including transparent gradients and lines.

Open the file 'transparency.ppt' in PowerPoint 2002. The first slide is titled 'Transparency'. Click on the Oval tool on the bottom toolbar and draw an oval (circle) anywhere on the slide. Select the circle, click the small black arrow next to the Fill Color icon on the lower toolbar and select 'More Fill Colors'. Notice the transparency slider at the bottom of the window. You can adjust the transparency level using this slider by typing in a number or using the top and bottom arrows next to the percentage (Fig. 19.11). Choose any percentage and click 'OK' to apply to the circle.

Along with single color transparency, you can also change transparency levels for gradient fills. Select the circle again, click the small black arrow next to the Fill Color icon and select 'Fill Effects'. In the Fill Effects window, click the radio button for 'Two colors'. Choose two distinctly different colors for 'Color 1' and 'Color 2'. Next, change the transparency levels for each color using the sliders in the center of the window (Fig. 19.12). Click 'OK' to apply the changes.

To get a better sense of transparency in PowerPoint, make a few copies of the circle, change their sizes and overlap them.

! ! ! ! ! ! ! ! ! ! ! ! ! ! ! ! ! ! Tip !   Hold down the 'Ctrl' key, click on an object and drag to make a copy.

Figure 19.11
Adjust the Fill Color
Transparency.

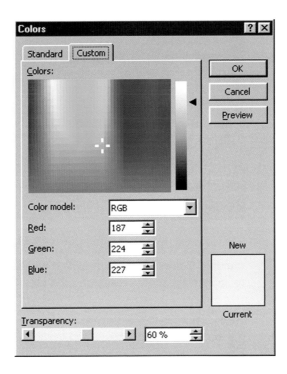

Figure 19.12
Two different colors, different
transparency settings.

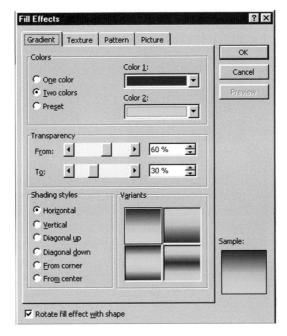

Take one or two of the circles and change the gradient colors, the
transparency settings, and the gradient direction (Fig. 19.13).

Select one of your circles, open the 'Line Styles' pop-up menu from the
bottom toolbar and change the line weight to '4½pts'. With the circle still
selected, click on the small black arrow next to 'Line Color' and select 'More

184

Figure 19.13
Various gradient fills and transparency settings.

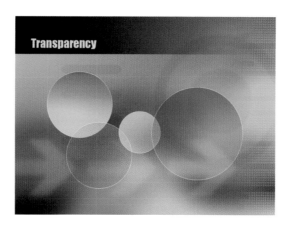

Line Colors' from the pop-up menu. Choose a very bold color from the standard Colors window and slide the transparency to about '80%'. Hit 'OK' to apply. Make similar changes to the other circles on your slide (Fig. 19.14).

Figure 19.14
Transparent circles with transparent outlines.

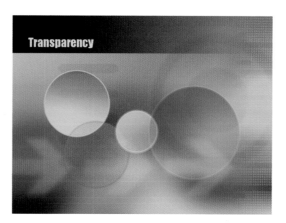

Transparency can even be applied to a picture-filled object. Select any one of your transparent circles, choose 'Fill Effects' from the Fill Color menu and click the Picture tab. Click 'Select Picture', navigate to the chapter folder on the CD, and choose 'syringe.jpg.' Click 'Insert' and 'OK' to apply. If you decide to change the transparency settings you can double-click the image and reset the transparency (Fig. 19.15). Save the PowerPoint file, giving it a name such as 'circles.ppt'.

Animation effects

In previous versions of PowerPoint, the animation effects were basic at best – you were limited to animating one object or group at a time; there wasn't a true 'dissolve ...' until now. With PowerPoint 2002, you have almost unlimited animation tools at your fingertips. And although we're not going to teach you everything about animating in PowerPoint (there's just too much), it is important to understand some new concepts before trying this out for yourself.

Figure 19.15
Transparent, picture-filled circle.

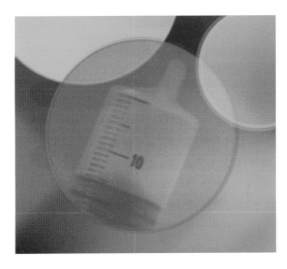

Figure 19.16
Custom Animation icon.

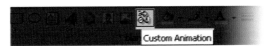

Open the file 'animation effects.ppt' from the chapter folder on the CD. Click the Custom Animation icon on the lower toolbar (Fig. 19.16). This will open the task pane on the right side of the screen. Press 'Play' at the bottom of the task pane to preview the slide animation.

The items in the Custom Animation list represent individual animation effects and not necessarily each object on the slide. You can apply as many effects as you want to any given object. The object 'Oval 5' has two effects, as you can see in the list.

You will also notice small, colored icons to the left of each item in the list. The green icons represent 'Entrance' effects. Apply any one of 52 effects to bring an object onto the slide. The yellow icons represent any one of 31 'Emphasis' effects. You can use these any time during the slide duration. The red icons represent 'Exit' effects. Use any of the 52 exit effects to animate an object off of the slide. A small path icon indicates 'Motion Paths' identical to the type of path you've chosen for the effect. There are 62 predefined motion paths to chose from, each fully editable, and if that's not enough you can also draw your own custom path.

You can reorder the list at will, using the arrows near the bottom of the task pane or by dragging and dropping the item(s) you wish to move. There are three 'Start' choices: 'On Click', 'With Previous', and 'After Previous'.

Right-click on any item in the list, or click on the small black arrow to the right of the item, to reveal the drop down menu. Select 'Show Advanced Timeline'. You will now see blue rectangles for each item in the effects list (Fig. 19.17). These rectangles represent the start and stop time for each effect, as well as the duration of the effect. You can drag either end of the rectangle to adjust animation timing, choose from five preset speeds, or type in a new speed (to 100th of a second) using decimal points. Reveal the 'Timing' window by selecting it from the drop down menu, accessible from any item in the list.

Figure 19.17
Advanced Timeline.

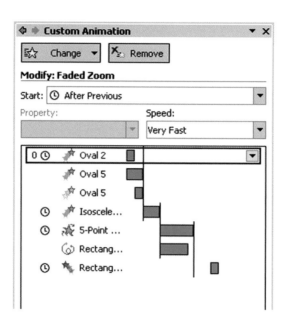

Click through each item in the list and you will notice that the top of the task pane changes. Depending on the type of effect you're using, this area will reveal property choices for the effect, such as: size, rotation, colors, etc. More 'Effect Options' can be edited from the drop down menu as well.

Rather than create a new slide to animate, let's begin by taking a few of the items in the animation list and change their effects and attributes.

Click on the first item in the list, 'Oval 2', and note that the 'Add Effect' button now reads 'Change'. Select Change > Entrance Effect > More Effects. Scroll down the list of entrance effects and try out a few for yourself. The effects are grouped in categories: basic, subtle, moderate, and exciting. As long as you have the 'Preview Effect' box checked, you can try out any of the effects before accepting the change.

Let's add an emphasis effect to the triangle. Select the triangle on the slide (not in the animation list). On the task pane, choose Add Effect > Emphasis Effects > More Effects > Spin. Change the 'Start' to 'With previous'. Reorder this effect so that it appears just above '5-point star 3'.

You can change the speed of the spin effect, the direction, and the amount of 'spin' you'd like, even to the exact degree. Click on the black arrow next to this list item to bring up the drop-down menu and select 'Effect Options'. Here you can program the spin to have a 'Smooth Start' or 'Smooth End' and 'Auto-reverse'.

So where and when will you use all of these new animation effects? The answer is: probably very rarely. Animation should be reserved for emphasizing key points, calling attention to important details, or possibly to introduce a presentation with an animated logo and title slide. It is bad practice to animate everything because your audience's attention will be drawn away from your important message. However, there are always exceptions, and great ways to work animation into your presentation. Open the file 'Animation Examples.ppt' from the chapter folder on the CD, choose 'read-only' when prompted, and hit the 'F5' key (or select Slide Show > View Show) to view the presentation.

Using images to keep the audience's attention

All too often, medical teachers use wordy slides or bullet points to explain concepts when the visual power of images will work better. Open the PowerPoint presentation 'Using Images' from the chapter folder on the CD. Hit 'F5' to view the Slide Show. The first slide is a simple bullet point list – pretty common stuff for medical educators.

Now look at the next few slides and imagine that you were giving this talk and wanted to draw out the issues surrounding each bullet point. We hope that you agree that using images rather than text is more attractive and memorable.

To duplicate this technique for yourself, open the file 'New.ppt' in the chapter folder. For this exercise you can use any template, and indeed any image – you may want to use some of your own. Just adjust the text accordingly.

Before you begin, make sure 'Snap to Grid' is turned on ('Ctrl G,' select 'Snap objects to grid'). Next, you will draw a perfect square with rounded corners. Select Autoshapes > Basic Shapes > Rounded Rectangle from the menu at the lower left of the screen. Position the cross-hair on the slide, hold down the 'Shift' key (to constrain proportions), and draw your first shape. We do not want the shape to have an outline for this exercise. Select the new shape, click the black arrow next to 'Line Color' on the bottom menu bar, and choose 'No Line' from the pop-up menu.

With your shape still selected, hold down the 'Ctrl' key (to duplicate) and 'Shift' key (to constrain horizontal or vertical) and then drag another identical box to the right. You now have two identical boxes.

Select both boxes, either by dragging a selection box around them both or by holding the 'Shift' key while you click each one. Now you will duplicate these two boxes for a total of four. Hold down the 'Ctrl' and 'Shift' keys and drag downward. Try to keep the vertical spacing between the boxes (gaps) similar to the horizontal space. Using the 'Snap objects to grid' option makes this much easier to accomplish.

Next, you will fill each box with an image from the CD. Double-click the first box then click the black arrow to the right of the 'Color' box. Select 'Fill Effects', 'Picture', 'Select Picture', and navigate to the chapter folder on the CD. Choose 'Informal.jpg' as your first image. Be sure to check the 'Lock picture aspect ratio' box. Select 'OK' twice.

Select the second box, fill this with the image 'OpRoom.jpg'; fill the third box with 'Structure.jpg', and the fourth box with 'Simulator.jpg'.

When all four boxes are filled, save your presentation.

Select Insert > Duplicate Slide. On this new slide, change the title to 'Informal teaching'. Hold the 'Shift' key and click to select the second, third, and fourth image boxes (not our first 'Informal teaching' image.) Choose Format > Autoshape from the top menu bar, slide the Transparency slider to '75%', and hit 'OK.'

Holding the 'Ctrl' key, click and drag a copy of the first image-filled box. Now, you want to position this duplicate a snap or two up and to the left of the original box (Fig. 19.18).

Figure 19.18
Position duplicate box a 'snap'
or two away from the original
(photography by Royal College
of Surgeons Photographic
Studios).

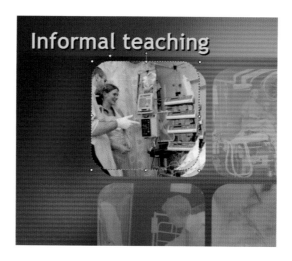

Hold the 'Shift' key, then click and drag the lower right handle to scale this box so that it covers about 75% of the other three boxes (Fig. 19.19).

Figure 19.19
Scale the duplicate to cover 75%
of the other three images
(photography by Royal College
of Surgeons Photographic
Studios).

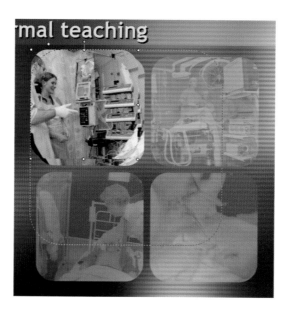

With the box selected, click the 'Shadow Style' icon on the lower menu bar. Choose 'Shadow Style 6' and release the mouse button. The shadow should default to transparent black.

Now, you will apply an animation effect to this larger image. Right-click on the large box and select 'Custom Animation'. In the Custom Animation task pane on the right, select Add Effect > Entrance > Faded Zoom.

!!!!!!!!!!!!!!!!!!!! Note !   If you do not see 'Faded Zoom' in the first list of recently used entrance effects, select 'More Effects' and choose 'Faded Zoom' from the Subtle category.

Near the top of the task pane, note the default Start setting is 'On Click'. Click this and change to 'Start: With Previous'. Change the Speed setting to 'Fast'. Hit the 'Play' button at the bottom of the task pane to preview the animation. Save your work.

Choose Insert > Duplicate Slide and change the title to 'In the operating room'. Double-click the small image box on the top right and slide the Transparency to '0%'. Now, you need to change the large image. Double-click the large box, click the black arrow next to 'Color,' choose 'Fill Effects', 'Picture', and then 'Select Picture'. Double-click on the file 'OpRoom.jpg' and hit 'OK' twice. With the large box still selected, hit the right arrow key (about 12 times or so) to move it just beyond the right of your smaller images. Double-click on the small, first image box and change the Transparency to '75%'.

Insert another duplicate slide and change the title to 'On structured courses'. Double-click the third image box (lower left) and change the transparency to '0%'. Double-click the large image and change the picture fill to 'Structure.jpg'. Move this large box over to cover the lower left, smaller box. You can use your mouse to drag it over, or the arrow keys if you prefer. Try to keep the distance from the smaller image similar to the previous slides. Double-click the small box on the top right and change the Transparency to '75%'.

Insert the last duplicate slide. Change the title to 'Using simulators'.

Double-click the small box in the lower right corner and change the Transparency to '0%'. Highlight the large box and change the picture fill to 'Simulator.jpg' and then move this large box to cover the lower right corner. Double-click on the small box in the lower left corner and change the Transparency to '75%'.

Save your presentation and then hit the 'F5' key to view the results.

Designing a poster

Julie Terberg

Quite often, a poster will be used for presenting purposes instead of an electronic slide show. It is fairly simple to use PowerPoint® to create the poster design and in this chapter we give you some guidelines to help you create an attractive and effective poster.

Gathering materials and information

Approach your poster layout as you would a presentation, beginning with information and image gathering. You might have digital images you want to use – a logo, charts or graphs, etc. Determine exactly what you want to accomplish with your poster and list the elements necessary to complete your layout. If you are scanning images, remember to scan them at approximately the same size as they will appear on the poster.

Determine poster size and orientation

Your poster will ultimately need to be printed in a large format size. These sizes vary greatly and it is always best to double-check the available sizes with the person who will be doing your printing. You might be directed to use a specific poster size or you could ask a colleague for advice and resources on sizes and printers. Posters come in many different sizes: 30×40 inches, 36×56 inches, 48×96 inches, and so on.

As well as choosing your final poster size, you will need to determine which page orientation – landscape or portrait – works better for the information you are assembling (you might be directed to use a specific orientation and size). It helps to begin by sketching your poster layout on paper. Divide your poster into two or three columns, much like a newspaper or magazine. Use simple blocks or outlines to indicate the approximate size for each of the elements to be included. This layout sketch will make it easier for you to begin developing the poster in PowerPoint. After creating a few layout sketches you might find that either landscape or portrait will work for your poster and the orientation will just be a matter of personal choice (Fig. 20.1).

Figure 20.1
Poster layout sketch.

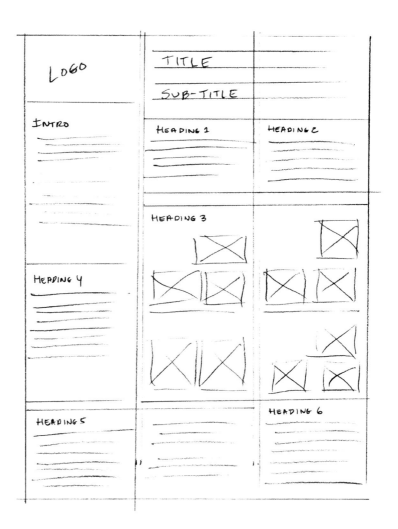

Page Set-up

Begin your poster design by defining the page size in PowerPoint. Select File > Page Setup, choose Slides sized for: Custom, type in the dimensions of your final poster size, and select 'Portrait' or 'Landscape' orientation.

!!!!!!!!!!!!!!!!!! Note !   PowerPoint has a page-size limitation of 56 inches (142.24 cm). If the final poster dimensions (either width or height) will exceed 56 inches, work at half size. Use 50% of the final width and height to determine the page dimensions in PowerPoint. For instance, if you will be printing a 48 × 96-inch poster, use 24 × 48 inches (60.96 × 121.92 cm) for your page set-up.

!!!!!!!!!!!!!!!!!! Note !   Remember to have the final poster printed at 200%!

To follow along with our example, change the page setup to 30 × 40 inches (76.2 × 101.6 cm), portrait orientation.

Slide Master

Now that you have defined the size of your blank canvas, it's time to start developing a template. If you set up the Slide Master properly, you will have a template that you can use over again for future posters.

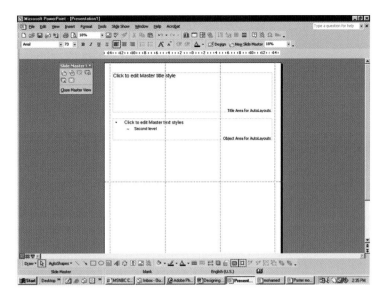

Figure 20.2
Guidelines set up to form three columns.

Select View > Master > Slide Master. You should see the default slide master set-up, with the title and text placeholders, as well as placeholders for date, footer, and page numbers. Select and delete the bottom three placeholders, as you will not need them for your poster design.

Notice the size of the title and text placeholders; the text is a bit too large for the amount of information we need to fit on our poster. Select the title placeholder; change the size to about '60 pts' and change the alignment to 'left'. With the placeholder selected, choose Format > Placeholder and click the 'Text Box' tab. Change the text anchor point to 'Top' and change each of the internal margins to '0'. Click 'OK'.

Select the first bulleted level in the text placeholder and change the text size to 60 pts; change the second level to 48 pts. Select and delete the remaining levels because it is highly unlikely that you will need more than two bullet levels for your poster. Select the placeholder outline and click and drag the center bottom point upwards. This will make the placeholder smaller and easier to work with. Save your file, giving it a name such as 'blankposter.ppt'.

Guidelines set-up

Following the layout sketches that you developed, position guidelines to define the columns and margins for your poster. Guidelines help you establish an ordered layout; keeping elements within a structure produces a more professional poster design. Type 'Ctrl G,' check the boxes for 'Snap objects to grid', and 'Display drawing guides on screen', and click 'OK'. Drag the vertical guideline to the left and position it at 14 inches (35.56 cm) or about 1 inch from the left edge. Hold down the 'Ctrl' key and drag a copy of this vertical guideline to the same distance from the right side of the page. Other vertical guidelines can be added in this same manner; the number will depend on how many columns you need. To follow our example layout, hold the 'Ctrl' key and drag a guideline to 4.67 inches (11.85 cm) from the left of center, and another 4.67 inches to the right of center. This will establish three columns for your poster design (Fig. 20.2).

Drag the horizontal guideline and position it about an inch from the top edge. Hold-down the 'Ctrl' key, drag a copy, and position this the same distance from the bottom edge to define the lower margin. As you continue to develop your poster design, you can add more guidelines if you want. PowerPoint will allow a maximum of eight horizontal and eight vertical guidelines. Save your work.

Logo placement

If you have a logo for your poster, place it in the top left or right corner of the slide master. Choose Insert > Picture > From File and select your logo file. Position the logo properly using the guides for placement. Remember to scale and optimize your logo prior to inserting it in PowerPoint. Our example includes the Queens University Belfast logo. After positioning the logo, you will need to scale and reposition the title placeholder on the slide master. Select the title placeholder and use the 'handles' on the sides to resize the text box (Fig. 20.3). Save your PowerPoint file again (remember to save often to avoid the hassle of recreating a lot of work).

Figure 20.3
Scale and reposition the Title placeholder.

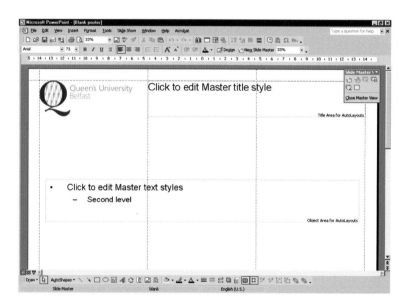

Vertical poster example

To give you a better understanding of how to approach your poster design, we're going to show you an original poster example and discuss the steps involved in redesigning the poster to make it more effective. This first poster was developed for the Department of Surgery at Queens University in Belfast (Fig. 20.4).

The original poster is set up for an A4 page size (7.5 × 10.83 inches, 19.05 × 27.52 cm). The background is filled with a pale yellow color. Guidelines are in place to establish three columns and five rows. Text and scanned graphs are positioned within the blocks of the layout grid.

Take a look at the redesigned poster and notice the changes to the consistency and clarity of the entire piece (Fig. 20.5).

Figure 20.4
Original vertical poster design.

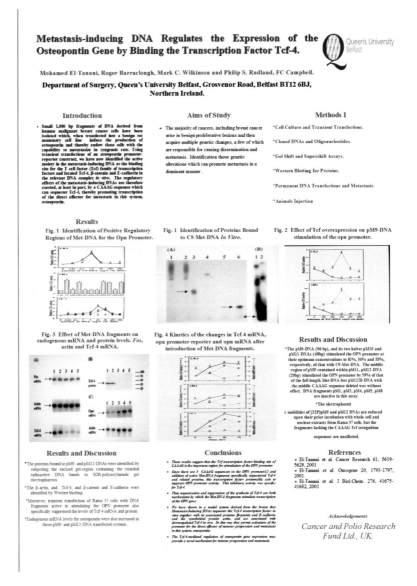

The first step in redesigning this poster was to change the page setup to 30 × 40 inches (76.2 × 01.6 cm). Because so much of the original poster was changing, it was easier to work with a new template (same attributes as 'blankposter.ppt' described in this chapter).

On the original poster, the Queens University Belfast logo is improperly scaled and does not appear in its correct proportions. We have already repositioned a properly scaled version of this logo onto the slide master in the 'blankposter' file.

The title was formatted and repositioned next. We chose to replace all of the poster fonts with Tahoma, a sans serif font that is very legible in different sizes. A deep red color was chosen to match the Queens University logo. We selected a left alignment for the title placeholder, changed the size to 60 pts

Figure 20.5
Redesigned poster.

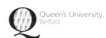

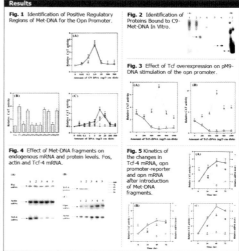

and decreased the line spacing to 0.95 lines. On the original poster, the subtitle and address were included in the same text block as the title. We separated this into a new text object, changed the alignment and sizes, and selected the warm gray color from the logo to use for the address.

The next task was to group elements together and to determine an effective layout. The 'Introduction' is set apart from the rest of the text by using an italic font. The 'Aims of Study' and 'Methods I' are placed in a light gray rectangle at the top of the poster, and 'Conclusions' are placed in a similar rectangle at the bottom.

The most dramatic difference in the revised poster is the 'Results' section. The word 'Results' is reversed out of a dark red rectangle and the entire section is bordered with a red line. A thin gray line separates each of the result figures. In the original poster, each of the charts and images was squashed to fit a specific size. Each one of these elements has been reformatted to its original proportions and using Photoshop®, all images have been improved for high contrast and legibility.

Overall, the text sizes are consistent. The font choices and colors are consistent and reflect the colors in the Queens University logo. All text blocks and graphic elements are aligned within the grid structure. The light colored rectangles and the bordered 'Results' area help to separate the different sections of the poster, making it much easier to focus on one area of information before moving on to the rest.

Try using some of these techniques for your next poster design. Use guidelines to set up the structure of your poster, group like information together, keep fonts and sizes consistent, and use borders and filled rectangles to separate different sections of information. These simple steps can help you design a great-looking and effective poster.

Chapter 21

Interactive teaching

Julie Terberg

Most presentations are delivered in a linear fashion: slide one is followed by slide two, which is followed by slide three, and so on. This works well when giving a stand-up presentation with little audience participation. You can, however, program your presentation in a non-linear way and use it as an interactive teaching tool. What do we mean by this?

With PowerPoint®open, locate the file called 'The Learning Curve.ppt' from the chapter folder on the CD. You will be prompted with a Password dialogue box. Click 'Read Only' to open the file and then hit the 'F5' key to view the Slide Show. Because the file is password protected, you will not be able to modify or save the file with another name.

Go ahead, put down the book and take 'The Learning Curve' interactive quiz.

How did you do? We hope you had a little fun with it.

This quiz was developed to show you some of the features that can be incorporated into an interactive presentation. This quiz includes a lot of animation; you might choose to begin with a simpler design.

Preparing your quiz

Before you begin creating your presentation in PowerPoint, you need to develop the quiz content. Determine how many questions you will ask, and how many answers for each question. Will you be varying the number of answers?

! ! ! ! ! ! ! ! ! ! ! ! ! ! ! ! ! ! ! Tip ! If you keep this number the same, you will have an easier time developing your slides.

Timing is important as well. Consider how much time it will take someone to complete the entire quiz.

Proofread all of your questions and answers, and make sure the wording is easily understandable. Short and to the point works best.

Assemble and resize any digital images you want to add to your slides. Perhaps you have an image for each question, or to add interest to any explanatory text (as in 'The Learning Curve' quiz).

Select your PowerPoint design template. It could be a template that you are currently using or you might have designed a new template following the instructions in Chapter 6; alternatively, select a template from the 'Templates' folder on the CD.

Navigation structure

When all of your questions and answers are completed, decide how you want the quiz to flow. You will probably want to include an opening slide to introduce the quiz. Like 'The Learning Curve' example, you might also decide to include a slide explaining how the quiz works.

Go through each set of answers and vary the position for each correct answer so as not to be too predictable. Decide what convention you will use to divide your answers: A, B, C, D; 1, 2, 3, 4; none of these, or maybe something unique. Will you include an explanatory slide after each question? Will you divide your questions into levels of difficulty, or sets?

It might help to sketch a quick diagram outlining the navigation for each slide; it can be as simple as a pencil sketch or a note after each answer in your electronic file (Fig. 21.1). Each question (with x possible answers) resides on its own slide. Next, for each question, we have included a 'wrong answer' slide, and a 'correct answer' slide. You can take this as far as you like, such as including a slide for each incorrect answer that will bounce the reader back

Figure 21.1
Quiz outline with navigation notes.

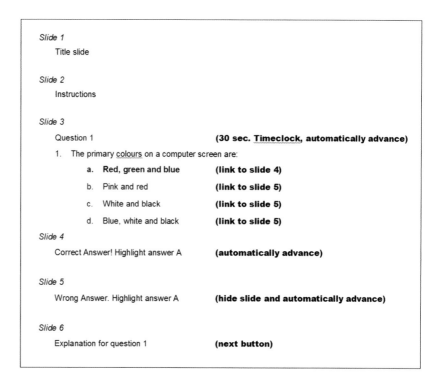

to the question. In our navigation structure, the 'wrong answer' slide and the 'correct answer' slide both navigate directly to the explanatory slide. From the explanatory slide, the user can click the 'next' button to advance to a new question. The quiz ends with a 'rate yourself' slide, and then a closing slide.

Developing slides in PowerPoint

Now that you have a plan, you can begin creating all of your slides in PowerPoint. After you create your 'introductory' or 'title' slide, and the 'quiz instructions' slide, design your first question slide. Decide how you are going to include question numbers, either by simply including the number before the question, or somewhere else on the slide.

If you haven't already done so, select View > Grid and Guides and check the box for 'Snap objects to grid'. Using the snap to grid function makes it much easier to draw and align objects on your slides.

Next, you need to draw a rectangle for each possible answer. This could be any graphic shape, with any possible outline or fill combination of your choice. Any graphic element or text item can be programed to work with links. Remember that legibility is important, so try not to get too complicated. Alternatively, you can select Autoshapes > Action Buttons and choose the first, blank button. Click and drag a rectangular button on the slide. You will be prompted with the 'Action Settings' dialogue box. Click 'Cancel' to close this window for now, as you will use this function for programing later. Select your 'button' (even if you have drawn a shape) and format it until you are satisfied with the design. Edit the fill color, fill effect, outline, or shadow to complement your design template.

With the button selected, click the 'Text Box' tool from the bottom menu bar and click on the button to begin adding text (or simply right-click, and choose 'Add text'). Type your first possible answer in this text box. Format the text to suit your design, including font, color choice, size, and shadow, if desired.

Now that your first answer is formatted, hold down the 'Ctrl' key, click this first answer button and drag to the right to make a copy. Select both buttons; hold 'Ctrl' and drag downward to make two more copies (Fig. 21.2). If you need more answer buttons, keep copying in this fashion until you have

Figure 21.2
Hold 'Ctrl' key and drag to duplicate buttons.

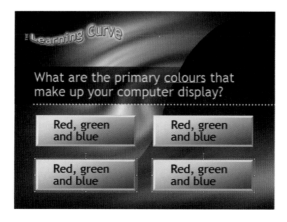

enough. You can always resize your buttons and use the 'Align or distribute' tools to even everything up.

Edit the answers to complete your first question slide. Remember to save your file often ('Ctrl S').

Next, select Insert > Duplicate Slide. This will be your 'correct answer' slide. Hold the 'Shift' key and select all three of your wrong answers. You will now edit the fill color, outline, and text color to make the wrong answers appear subdued on the slide. This usually means selecting a darker color when working on a dark-colored template, or a lighter color on a light-colored template. Doing so will make your correct answer stand out on the slide (Fig. 21.3).

Figure 21.3
Wrong answers subdued to highlight correct answer.

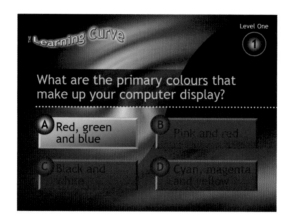

You might wish to include a shape with the words 'correct' or 'you're right', or other words of your choice (Fig. 21.4).

Figure 21.4
'You're right!' builds onto the slide.

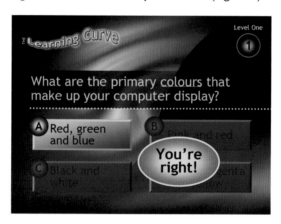

After your 'correct answer' slide is finished, select Insert > Duplicate Slide. On this new slide, select the shape with 'correct' or 'right' answer and edit the text to say 'incorrect, try again' or 'the right answer is ... ' Save your file (Fig. 21.5).

The next step is to create the first explanatory slide. This is optional and is used to give a short rationale for the correct answer to the question. It helps the quiz-taker understand a little more about the question subject (Fig. 21.6). Save your file.

Figure 21.5
'The correct answer is …'
builds onto the slide.

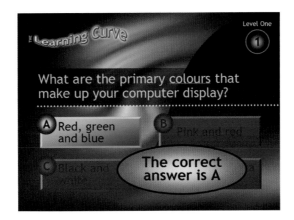

Figure 21.6
Explanatory slide.

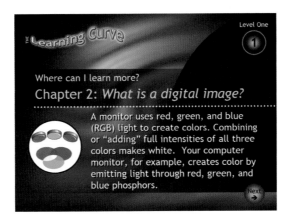

You have now completed a set of slides for the first question; we'll get to programming the quiz a little later.

Select View > Slide Sorter to see a thumbnail version of all of your slides. Select the first question slide, type 'Ctrl C' to copy and then insert the cursor after the last slide and type 'Ctrl V' to paste.

Select this new slide and choose View > Normal. Edit the text to reflect your next question and all answers. Duplicate the slide (Insert > Duplicate Slide).

Pick-up and apply

Now that you have already formatted the look of your subdued 'wrong answer' buttons, it's easy to pick-up the style and apply it to your new slide. If you followed the instructions in Chapter 7, you already know how to use the eye-dropper tools and have added them to your toolbar. If you don't have a clue what we're talking about, go back to Chapter 7 and follow the instructions for 'Pick-up and Apply'.

With the eye-droppers in easy reach on the toolbar, hit the 'Page Up' key a few times to go back to the first 'you're right!' slide. Select one of the subdued wrong answer buttons and click the 'Pick Up Object Style' icon (eye-dropper). Next, go to your new 'you're right!' slide, hold the 'Shift' key down, select all of the wrong answer buttons and click the 'Apply Object

Style' icon (other eye-dropper). This 'style' will remain in memory ready to apply to another object until you pick up another style (or exit the program).

If you created a shape for your first question that says 'you're right' or something similar, go back to that slide and copy the shape to the clipboard ('Ctrl C'). Navigate to your new 'you're right!' slide again, and type 'Ctrl V' to paste.

!!!!!!!!!!!!!!!!!! Tip !   If you want this shape to animate onto the slide, program the custom animation the first time the shape appears and then copy it to your subsequent slides. The animation will be copied along with the shape.

Insert another duplicate slide, delete the 'you're right!' shape, go back to your first 'the correct answer is ...' or 'wrong answer' slide, copy the shape and paste it onto this slide.

Now that you understand how to copy and edit the question-and-answer slides, as well as the explanatory slides, you can go ahead and create the rest of the slides for your quiz.

Programing hyperlinks

A hyperlink is a connection from one slide to another slide, a custom show, a web page, or a file. The hyperlink itself can be text or an object such as a picture, graph, shape, or WordArt®. You will assign a hyperlink to each of your answer buttons to direct the quiz taker to the proper slide for each answer. This allows you to program the quiz to jump from one slide to another, backwards or forwards in the slide sequence.

Go to your first question slide, select the first answer and choose Slide Show > Action Settings (or right-click and choose 'Action Settings' or 'Hyperlink'). In the Action Settings dialogue box, click the radio button for 'Hyperlink to', scroll down the drop-down menu and select 'Slides' (Fig. 21.7).

Figure 21.7
Action Settings dialogue box.

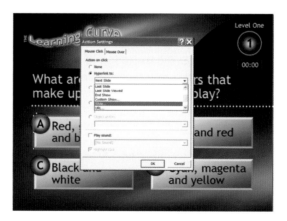

Now, determine whether this answer is correct or incorrect and choose the appropriate slide that you want the user to see when they select this answer (Fig. 21.8). Click 'OK' and then 'OK' again to close the 'Action Settings' dialogue box. That's it: you have programed a hyperlink. Continue to do this for all of your answer boxes; carefully selecting the hyperlink slides so that you are linking to the proper slide.

Figure 21.8
Hyperlink to Slide dialogue box.

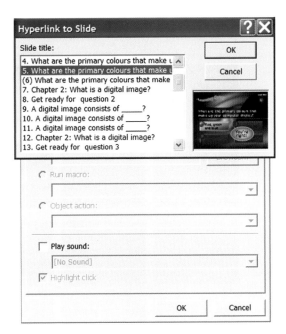

Hiding slides

If you are following the structure of 'The Learning Curve' quiz, you will have a question slide, a 'correct answer' slide, a 'wrong answer' slide, and an explanatory slide for each question in the quiz. To prevent the quiz-taker seeing the 'wrong answer' slide directly after they have chosen the right answer, you need to 'Hide' all of the wrong answer slides. This doesn't mean that they're gone forever; any buttons programed to advance to the hidden slides will still work and will, in fact, bring up the 'wrong answer' slides. When the quiz-taker sees the 'correct answer' slide, the quiz will just skip over the wrong answer and go directly to the explanatory slide.

Go to the Slide Sorter view (View > Slide Sorter), select the slide you want to hide, choose Slide Show > Hide Slide or right-click 'Hide Slide' (Fig. 21.9). Notice the slash mark over the slide number indicating the hidden slides. Follow this step to hide all of the wrong answer slides. Hold the 'Ctrl' key down if you want to select more than one slide at a time.

Slide timing

It's pretty simple to create a countdown clock for your question slides. Using the 'Text Box' tool, type in your starting number. The example uses 00:30. If you want, you can add a border around the text. The important step is to fill the text box with a solid color so that as you add numbers, they will cover the previous one (makes programing much simpler). Hold down the 'Ctrl' key and drag a copy of the starting number (or 'Ctrl D' to duplicate). Edit the number to one second less than the first (example: 00:29) (Fig. 21.10).

With this number selected, choose Slide Show > Custom Animation. Click 'Add Effect' from the top of the task pane, then 'Entrance' and select a very simple effect, such as 'wipe' or 'fade', to animate the countdown.

Figure 21.9
Hide slides.

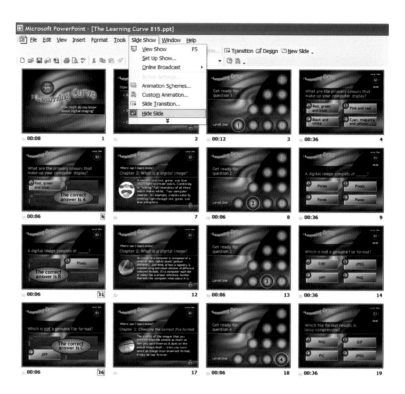

Figure 21.10
Duplicate first numbers for
time clock and edit by
one second.

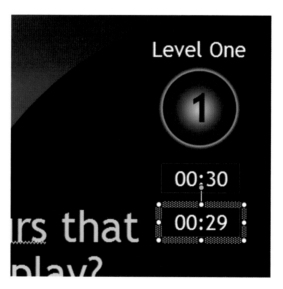

Next to 'Start', select 'After previous'. Right-click on this item in the task
pane list, select 'Timing', and change the 'Delay' to '1' second (Fig. 21.11).
    Now when you duplicate this number, the Entrance effect and timing will
be copied along with it. Edit the numbers, and continue duplicating and
editing until you have a text box for each second on the time clock. When
you are finished, drag a selection box around all of the time clock numbers

Figure 21.11
Edit the Timing to include
a 1-second delay.

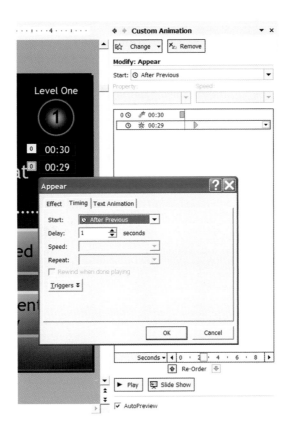

and use the 'Align and Distribute' tool to line them up right on top of one
another (Fig. 21.12). Click the 'Play' button at the bottom of the task pane to
see the time clock in action.

Figure 21.12
Use the Align tool to position
all numerals on top of
each other.

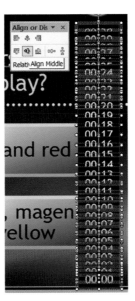

Automatic transitions

Of course, the time clock is useless if the slide is going to remain on the screen. You will need to program these slides to advance automatically to the next slide in the given number of seconds.

At the top of the task pane, select the small black arrow and choose 'Slide Transition' from the drop-down menu. Near the bottom of this task pane, notice the section for 'Advance Slide'. Uncheck the button for 'On mouse click' and check the radio button for 'Automatically after'. Change the number of seconds to reflect your time clock (Fig. 21.13).

Figure 21.13
Advance slide automatically.

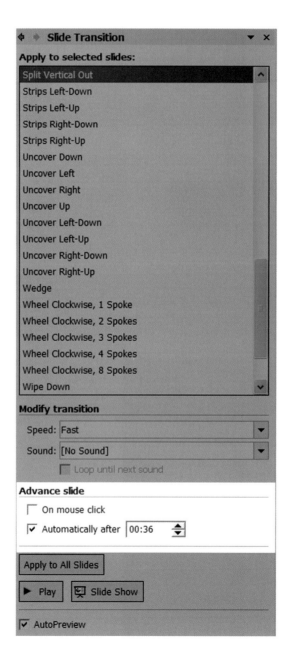

If you have programed any animation to occur on the slide prior to the time clock (either the question or the answer buttons) you will need to sum all of the seconds or half-seconds for these animations and add it to the total.

In 'The Learning Curve' quiz, the 'correct answer' and 'wrong answer' slides have been programed to advance automatically after 6 seconds. This gives the quiz-taker time to see the message, the correct answer, and move on to the explanation.

'Next' buttons

In 'The Learning Curve' quiz, you'll notice there are 'next' buttons at the bottom of each explanatory slide. These give the quiz-takers some direction, and let them know they have time to read the explanation before advancing to the next question. Use plain text or an action button and type in the word 'next' (or whatever you prefer). Follow the steps for programing hyperlinks above and program the 'next' button to navigate to the proper slide (if it will always be the next slide, you can choose this from the hyperlink menu). When you copy and paste this button on another slide, remember to re-program the hyperlink if necessary.

Prepare your quiz carefully, and check and recheck the hyperlinks to make sure the user will be directed to the proper slide. Have fun creating your own interactive quiz.

Chapter 22

Using the PowerPoint® templates on the CD

Julie Terberg

We have included 20 PowerPoint® templates in the chapter folder on the CD. You have purchased the rights to these templates for your own use. Please comply with our request to keep the templates in limited circulation. You cannot distribute them to friends, nor post them on the Internet. Refer to Chapter 6 for detailed instructions on designing your own templates.

The design template names give a very brief description of their content and appearance. You can customize any of the templates by adding a logo or by inserting accent photos.

Copying the templates to your system

Templates are named with the .pot suffix, as opposed to .ppt for a presentation file. You can open them from the CD or, for quicker access at a later date, you could copy all the templates to your hard drive. The default folder for Microsoft® templates is 'C:\Windows\Application Data\Microsoft\templates'. Create a new folder within this 'templates' folder and give it a name such as 'Medical templates'. Copy all of the .pot files from the CD into this folder to access from within PowerPoint.

Opening a template

There are a few ways you can work with the design templates. If you are using them for the first time you might want to view the slides that have been formatted with each template. Select File > Open and navigate to the folder containing the templates (either the 'templates' folder on the CD or the new folder if you copied them to your system). Select 'Preview' from the 'Views' icon at the top of your navigation window to see a small thumbnail version of each template.

When opening any of the design templates using this method, you will see five formatted slides. Each of the slides includes notes about what type of

Figure 22.1
Top left, sample title slide; top middle, sample text slide; top right, color palette slide; bottom left, sample print version title slide; bottom right, sample print version text slide.

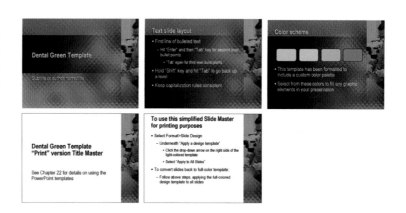

slide it is and how to use it (Fig. 22.1). The first slide is a sample title slide. The second slide is an example of a text slide. Replace the text on either slide, or delete them both and insert new slides with blank placeholders to work with. The third slide in each template set includes a sample color palette. Each design template has been formatted with a color scheme that complements the background image. Use these colors for graphics throughout your slides for a more consistent-looking presentation. Any charts or diagrams will be formatted using these four colors first. The fourth and fifth slides are examples of the 'print masters'. Slide 5 includes instructions for applying the 'print masters' to your entire presentation. The 'print masters' are simplified versions of the slide masters, allowing you to print a much quicker version of your presentation and save a lot of ink in the process.

Opening a blank template

Once you are familiar with the PowerPoint templates you might not need to view (and delete) the formatted slides and choose instead to begin with a blank presentation. With PowerPoint open, select File > New and choose 'From Design Template' on the 'New Presentation' task pane (Fig. 22.2). When the task pane changes to 'Slide Design', select 'Browse' and open up your new folder 'Medical templates'. Again, to see a thumbnail version of each template, click on the 'Views' icon near the top of the window and select 'Preview' from the drop down menu. Select a template and click 'Apply'.

Apply a design template to an existing presentation

You might already have a completed presentation and just want to change the design template. Open the existing presentation in PowerPoint and then select Format > Slide Design. On the slide design task pane click 'Browse' and navigate to the folder containing the new template you want to apply. Select your new design and then choose 'Apply'. If you choose any of the templates from the CD you will be prompted with a window stating that the template has multiple slide masters and asking you if you want to copy the other masters into your presentation for later use. Select 'Yes'. This will copy the print masters into your presentation.

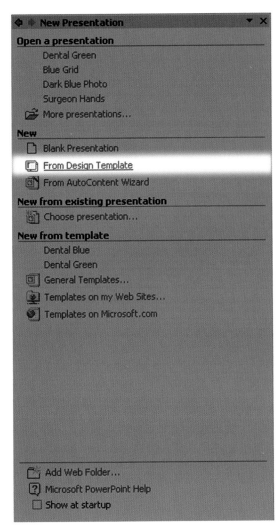

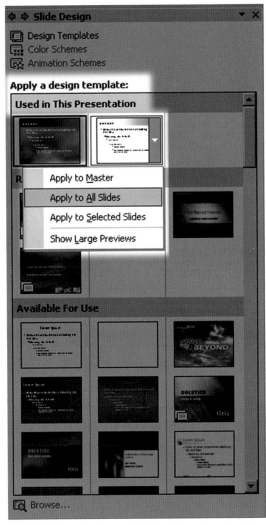

Figure 22.2 Select 'From a Design Template' on the task pane.

Figure 22.3 Applying the 'Print Master' to all slides.

Applying the print masters

To apply the print masters to your presentation select Format > Slide Design. Below 'Apply a design template', click the drop-down arrow next to the right side of the light-colored template and select 'Apply to All Slides' (Fig. 22.3). Your presentation will be updated to reflect the lighter slide masters. You can save this version of your presentation if you want, or simply select Edit > Undo, or type 'Ctrl Z' to go back to the full color version. If you made the mistake of saving over your original file, just repeat the process of changing the Slide Design, only select the full color Slide Master instead and 'Apply to All Slides'.

Inserting a logo

In most cases, it is best to have a logo 'float' on the background by inserting a .png file on the slide masters. The .png file allows transparency and, if created properly, your logo will have a nice, smooth edge instead of a raggedy, pixilated edge. Chapter 3 contains detailed instructions for creating a transparent background in Photoshop Elements®.

When you are ready to insert a logo, select View > Masters > Slide Master. Next, choose Insert > Picture > From File, and navigate to the folder containing your logo. Either double-click on the file or select the logo file and click 'Insert'. Click and drag the logo to move it into position. Where should you put it? This will depend on the design of both logo and template. Generally, the logo will work best in the upper right, lower left, or lower right corner (Fig. 22.4).

Figure 22.4
Position logo on the
Slide Master.

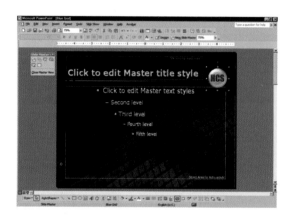

After you place the logo in position, you'll need to copy it to the other slide masters. Select the logo, type 'Ctrl C' (copy), advance to the next master and type 'Ctrl V' (paste). Continue pasting the logo on each slide master. You might want to make the logos slightly larger on the title masters.

Inserting photos on the slide masters

You can embellish most of the design templates by adding or replacing photos on the slide masters. Take a look at the design template called 'Dental Blue'. Three dental images have been inserted on each of the slide masters. You can replace these images to customize the template for another medical theme, or use this design as inspiration to customize another template by adding images in the same manner.

To replace the images on the 'Dental Blue' template or similar design templates, select View > Master > Slide Master. Hold down the shift key, click on all three images to select them and hit 'Delete'. Notice the three soft shadows on the background: use them as a guide to place your new images. Your new images should be sized to approximately 125 × 85 pixels to match the original dental images. Select Insert > Picture > From File, navigate to the folder containing your sized images, and insert one at a time. Eyeball the position for each of the three new images and then use the 'Align or Distribute' tools for accuracy (Draw > Align or Distribute > Align Top and then 'Distribute Horizontally').

Saving your revised templates

When you are satisfied with the revisions you have made to the design template, you will need to save it with a new name. Select File > Save As, choose 'Design Template' from the 'Save as type' drop down menu and type in a descriptive name for your design. Remember to save the templates in a folder that you can access later, either the default template folder (C:\Windows\Application Data\Microsoft\templates) or another folder of your choice.

Chapter 23

PowerPoint® and Photoshop Elements® shortcuts

Julie Terberg

As a beginner, it is a good idea to navigate through the menu systems of both of these powerful programs to familiarize yourself with their structure. As you get accustomed to them, you will want to begin using shortcuts. These simple, and often intuitive, keystrokes allow you to apply complex commands much more rapidly, because they avoid you having to reach for that pesky rodent.

Many of the shortcuts have been outlined already as you have worked through the chapters. We cannot list all the shortcuts here, there are just too many, but we have tried to include the most useful ones for each program.

We have also included a .pdf of the shortcuts on the CD and on the website. You can use this to print off a poster for your office or print it on a mouse mat. Most large stationery stores will do this for you, or you can search online using the terms print and mouse mats to find suppliers in your country.

PowerPoint shortcuts

You can find a list of all of the PowerPoint® shortcuts in the PowerPoint help menu, search for keyboard shortcuts (Tables 23.1 and 23.2).

Table 23.1   These commands are useful when preparing your slides

Command	Keystroke
Insert duplicate slide	Ctrl + D
Draw a perfect circle, square or line (constrain proportions)	Hold Shift key while drawing object
Change capitalization of text	Highlight text and click Shift + F3. Keep repeating to scroll through ALL CAPS, Initial Caps and all lower case
Insert ©	Type (c) (Works in Word as well)
Insert ™	Type (TM) (Works in Word as well)
Insert®	Type (R) (Works in Word as well)
Make text superscript	Highlight text and type Ctrl + + (plus) sign
Make text subscript	Highlight text and type Ctrl + = (equal) sign
Remove super- or sub-script	Ctrl + space bar
View guides	Ctrl + G
Delete a word	Ctrl + backspace
Undo	Ctrl + Z
Bold	Ctrl + B
Italicize	Ctrl + I
Select all	Ctrl + A (selects all objects in Normal View, or all slides in Slide Sorter View)
Copy	Ctrl + C
Paste	Ctrl + V
Save	Ctrl + S
Print	Ctrl + P
Move an object	Select the object and use arrow keys to move in any direction OR click to select object and keep mouse button depressed while dragging object to new position

Table 23.2   These commands are useful when you are showing your slide show

Command	Keystroke
Start slide show	F5
Go to first slide	1 + enter
Next slide or animation on this slide	Enter, N, page down, right arrow (>) or space bar
Previous slide or animation on this slide	P, page up, left arrow (<) or back space
Go to a slide by name	Right-click>go>by title or Right-click>go>slide navigator
Go to any slide	'n' + enter, where n = the number of the slide
Show black slide	B or period (full stop)
Go back to normal slide	B or period (full stop again)
Show white slide	W or comma
Go back to normal slide	W or comma again or hold down both mouse buttons for 2 seconds
Show shortcuts during a slide show	F1
Hide or show arrow pointer	A
Erase drawing on slide	E
Change pointer to pen	Ctrl + P
Change pointer to arrow	Ctrl + A
Hide pointer or pen	Ctrl + H
Show speaker notes	Right-click>speaker notes
End show	Escape

Photoshop Elements shortcuts

Note that many of these commands are the same in PowerPoint.

Table 23.3 These commands are based on the file menu

Command	Keystroke
New	Ctrl + N
Open	Ctrl + O
Save	Ctrl + S
Save As	Ctrl + Shift + S
Close	Ctrl + W
Close Photoshop Elements	Ctrl + Q
Print	Alt + Ctrl + P

Table 23.4
These commands are used when editing

Command	Keystroke
Cut	Ctrl + X
Undo	Ctrl + Z
Copy	Ctrl + C
Paste as new image	Ctrl + V
Paste as new layer	Ctrl + L
Paste as new selection	Ctrl + E
Fill with foreground color	Alt + backspace

Table 23.5
More general commands

Command	Keystroke
Zoom in	Ctrl + + (plus)
Zoom out	Ctrl + − (minus)
Fit on screen	Ctrl + 0 (zero)
Select all	Ctrl + A
Deselect	Ctrl + D
Adjust levels	Ctrl + L
Invert selection	Shift + Ctrl + I

Table 23.6
The following commands are used to select specific tools from the toolbox

Command	Keystroke
Paintbrush	B
Crop	C
Eraser	E
Gradient	G
Lasso	L
Dodge and Burn	O
Sharpen	P
Blur	R
Type	T
Move	V
Magic Wand	W
Zoom	Z

Index

ELSEVIER CD-ROM LICENCE AGREEMENT

Please read the following agreement carefully before using this product. This product is licensed under the terms contained in this licence agreement ('agreement'). By using this product, You, an individual or entity including employees, agents and representatives ('You' or 'Your'), acknowledge that You have read this agreement, that You understand it, and that You agree to be bound by the terms and conditions of this agreement. Elsevier Limited ('Elsevier') expressly does not agree to license this product to You unless You assent to this agreement. If You do not agree with any of the following terms, You may, within thirty (30) days after Your receipt of this product return the unused product and all accompanying documentation to Elsevier for a full refund.

DEFINITIONS As used in this Agreement, these terms shall have the following meanings:

'Proprietary Material' means the valuable and proprietary information content of this Product including without limitation all indexes and graphic materials and software used to access, index, search and retrieve the information content from this Product developed or licensed by Elsevier and/or its affiliates, suppliers and licensors.

'Product' means the copy of the Proprietary Material and any other material delivered on CD-ROM and any other human-readable or machine-readable materials enclosed with this Agreement, including without limitation documentation relating to the same.

OWNERSHIP This Product has been supplied by and is proprietary to Elsevier and/or its affiliates, suppliers and licensors. The copyright in the Product belongs to Elsevier and/or its affiliates, suppliers and licensors and is protected by the copyright, trademark, trade secret and other intellectual property laws of the United Kingdom and international treaty provisions, including without limitation the Universal Copyright Convention and the Berne Copyright Convention. You have no ownership rights in this Product. Except as expressly set forth herein, no part of this Product, including without limitation the Proprietary Material, may be modified, copied or distributed in hardcopy or machine-readable form without prior written consent from Elsevier. All rights not expressly granted to You herein are expressly reserved. Any other use of this Product by any person or entity is strictly prohibited and a violation of this Agreement.

SCOPE OF RIGHTS LICENSED (PERMITTED USES) Elsevier is granting to You a limited, non-exclusive, non-transferable licence to use this Product in accordance with the terms of this Agreement. You may use or provide access to this Product on a single computer or terminal physically located at Your premises and in a secure network or move this Product to and use it on another single computer or terminal at the same location for personal use only, but under no circumstances may You use or provide access to any part or parts of this Product on more than one computer or terminal simultaneously.

You shall not (a) copy, download, or otherwise reproduce the Product or any part(s) thereof in any medium, including, without limitation, online transmissions, local area networks, wide area networks, intranets, extranets and the Internet, or in any way, in whole or in part, except for printing out or downloading nonsubstantial portions of the text and images in the Product for Your own personal use; (b) alter, modify, or adapt the Product or any part(s) thereof, including but not limited to decompiling, disassembling, reverse engineering, or creating derivative works, without the prior written approval of Elsevier; (c) sell, license or otherwise distribute to third parties the Product or any part(s) thereof; or (d) alter, remove, obscure or obstruct the display of any copyright, trademark or other proprietary notice on or in the Product or on any printout or download of portions of the Proprietary Materials.

RESTRICTIONS ON TRANSFER This Licence is personal to You, and neither Your rights hereunder nor the tangible embodiments of this Product, including without limitation the Proprietary Material, may be sold, assigned, transferred or sublicensed to any other person, including without limitation by operation of law, without the prior written consent of Elsevier. Any purported sale, assignment, transfer or sublicense without the prior written consent of Elsevier will be void and will automatically terminate the Licence granted hereunder.

TERM This Agreement will remain in effect until terminated pursuant to the terms of this Agreement. You may terminate this Agreement at any time by removing from Your system and destroying the Product and any copies of the Proprietary

Material. Unauthorized copying of the Product, including without limitation, the Proprietary Material and documentation, or otherwise failing to comply with the terms and conditions of this Agreement shall result in automatic termination of this licence and will make available to Elsevier legal remedies. Upon termination of this Agreement, the licence granted herein will terminate and You must immediately destroy the Product and all copies of the Product and of the Proprietary Material, together with any and all accompanying documentation. All provisions relating to proprietary rights shall survive termination of this Agreement.

LIMITED WARRANTY AND LIMITATION OF LIABILITY Elsevier warrants that the software embodied in this Product will perform in substantial compliance with the documentation supplied in this Product, unless the performance problems are the result of hardware failure or improper use. If You report a significant defect in performance in writing to Elsevier within ninety (90) calendar days of Your having purchased the Product, and Elsevier is not able to correct same within sixty (60) days after its receipt of Your notification, You may return this Product, including all copies and documentation, to Elsevier and Elsevier will refund Your money. In order to apply for a refund on Your purchased Product, please contact the return address on the invoice to obtain the refund request form ('Refund Request Form'), and either fax or mail Your signed request and Your proof of purchase to the address indicated on the Refund Request Form. Incomplete forms will not be processed. Defined terms in the Refund Request Form shall have the same meaning as in this Agreement.

You understand that, except for the limited warranty recited above, Elsevier, its affiliates, licensors, third party suppliers and agents (together 'the suppliers') make no representations or warranties, with respect to the product, including, without limitation the proprietary material. All other representations, warranties, conditions or other terms, whether express or implied by statute or common law, are hereby excluded to the fullest extent permitted by law.

In particular but without limitation to the foregoing none of the suppliers make any representions or warranties (whether express or implied) regarding the performance of Your pad, network or computer system when used in conjunction with the product, nor that the product will meet Your requirements or that its operation will be uninterrupted or error-free.

Except in respect of death or personal injury caused by the suppliers' negligence and to the fullest extent permitted by law, in no event (and regardless of whether such damages are foreseeable and of whether such liability is based in tort, contract or otherwise) will any of the suppliers be liable to You for any damages (including, without limitation, any lost profits, lost savings or other special, indirect, incidental or consequential damages) arising out of or resulting from: (i) Your use of, or inability to use, the product; (ii) data loss or corruption; and/or (iii) errors or omissions in the proprietary material.

If the foregoing limitation is held to be unenforceable, our maximum liability to You in respect thereof shall not exceed the amount of the licence fee paid by You for the product. The remedies available to You against Elsevier and the licensors of materials included in the product are exclusive.

If the information provided In the Product contains medical or health sciences information, it is intended for professional use within the medical field. Information about medical treatment or drug dosages is intended strictly for professional use, and because of rapid advances in the medical sciences, independent verification of diagnosis and drug dosages should be made.

The provisions of this Agreement shall be severable, and in the event that any provision of this Agreement is found to be legally unenforceable, such unenforceability shall not prevent the enforcement or any other provision of this Agreement.

GOVERNING LAW This Agreement shall be governed by the laws of England and Wales. In any dispute arising out of this Agreement, You and Elsevier each consent to the exclusive personal jurisdiction and venue in the courts of England and Wales.

Minimum system requirements

Windows

Intel Pentium processor
Microsoft Windows 95 OSR 2.0, Windows 98 SE, Windows Millennium,
Windows NT1 4.0 with Service Pack 5, or Windows 2000
64 MB of RAM
24 MB of available hard-disk space

Macintosh

PowerPC processor
Mac OS software version 8.6, 9.0.4, or Mac OS X
64 MB of RAM
24 MB of available hard-disk space

Technical Support

Technical support for this product is available between 7:30 a.m. and 7 p.m. CST, Monday through Friday. Before calling, be sure that your computer meets the minimum system requirements to run this software. Inside the United States and Canada, call 1-800-692-9010. Inside the United Kingdom, call 0080069290100. Outside North America, call +1-314-872-8370.

You may also fax your questions to +1-314-997-5080, or contact Technical Support through e-mail: technical.support@elsevier.com.